NAPOLEON & I

OR

THE SIGNIFICANT MISS FANNY MITCHELL

BY

ROBERT SHELLEY

Quiller

Also by Robert Shelley

Flies in Paradise
[A romantic wander through some of the key events in the history of medicine]

For SMR

This edition published in the UK in 2011
by Quiller, an imprint of Quiller Publishing Ltd

British Library Cataloguing-in-Publication Data
A catalogue record for this book
is available from the British Library

ISBN 978 1 84689 114 4

Printed in Malta by Gutenberg Press Ltd

Quiller
An imprint of Quiller Publishing Ltd
Wykey House, Wykey, Shrewsbury, SY4 1JA
Tel: 01939 261616 Fax: 01939 261606
E-mail: info@quillerbooks.com
Website: www.countrybooksdirect.com

Contents

(Contents continued overleaf)

(Contents continued)

~1~
The Two Questions

I first met Napoleon rather a long time ago. It was in the little town of Laon just a few days after Waterloo. The Emperor (as he still was) had most certainly not been demoralized by the loss of the battle. It had merely been an annoying setback to his campaign which, if you take the broad sweep as he was bound to do, wasn't going all that badly considering how short a time it had been in operation. Already deep into plans for its continuation, and confident that all was not lost, he had written to brother Joseph in Paris: "But people must help me, not deafen me with advice." Yet advice, however unwelcome, was just about all the help he was going to get.

But what on earth was I doing in Laon? Ever since the Emperor had escaped from Elba I had been stationed in Paris as an observer. When the news of Blücher's defeat at Ligny reached us I decided off my own bat that my place was closer to the action than the hospitals of Paris, inspirational though they may have been with the likes of Laennec and Dupuytren working there. So north I went and couldn't believe my luck when I bumped into the Emperor heading south. What should I do? Here we had an emperor whose invincible Imperial Guard had not just retreated but been driven, panic stricken and disorganized, from the field. He evidently was not prepared to accept the reality of the situation. His future would be well worth keeping an eye on and that is precisely what I decided to do.

The critical turning point in his deliberations was his reception at Laon, for it was here that for the first time he came up against the power of Public Opinion. Politics was about to bring him down. However, as we enter this, the final stage, of Napoleon's life, it would be well to remember that events were about to take on a momentum of their own and as they progressed, medical aspects, administrative as well as clinical, began to enter the picture.

Regrettably, this has not been fully appreciated owing to a considerable lack of understanding, mostly of the significance of his clinical history and post-mortem report(s) but also of the circumstances of his captivity. The Establishment (subsection Napoleonic History) is not exactly enamoured with the re-writing of his medical history, particularly as it rocks the boat of received wisdom (damn near sinks it!). Moreover, delving into the records of the past is to enter the realms of historical writing – and these are as treacherous as the Bermuda Triangle where truth is swallowed leaving only the doodlings of man's imagination by way of an explanation.

The word treacherous, incidentally, was used by Hippocrates in a most unexpected context – though, if you think about it, it is relevant here. Its opening words are well known: "Life is short, the Art long," but not its continuation: "Opportunity fleeting, Experience treacherous, Judgment difficult." The 'Art' is, of course, medicine and even though Hippocrates did not mean *all* experience, it should make the proponents of evidence-based medicine sit up and think. Medicine is still an art, though some may find this difficult to believe. It is surrounded by science, but approach the bedside, the patient, and fail to treat it as an art at your peril (and the patient's!).

So, what went on in Napoleon's own special world between Waterloo and his death on St Helena? That depends on who you choose as your 'authority'. But so contradictory are the various sources – that's what keeps the industry going – that you feel dumped in the Triangle with no hope of rescue.

At the start of his *History of the Peloponnesian War*, Thucydides put the matter nice and succinctly: "My conclusions have cost me some labour from the want of coincidence between accounts of the same occurrences by different eyewitnesses, arising sometimes from imperfect memory, sometimes from undue partiality for one side or the other." And that was nearly two-and-a-half thousand years ago!

There is, however, one specialized source clamouring for attention and that is his medical record throughout those years. Tragically, it has serious trouble making its voice heard – just like the wretched Tithonus of Greek legend: Eos, the Greek Aurora, the Dawn, rejoiced in the affliction common to many female mythological characters: she could not resist a handsome young man. After a number of false starts she settled on Tithonus, half brother to Priam, king of Troy. Overwhelmed by passion she begged Zeus to grant him immortality. Zeus obliged. But immortality requires eternal youth if it is to be even halfway bearable, a point overlooked by Eos. When she could stand the sight of the ancient wrinkly no longer she shut him away in a room where only the faint crying of his trembling voice could be heard. Eventually the gods took pity on him and ended his misery by turning him into a cicada. (I wonder what the cicada thought about the deal? And poor Eos, she was not allowed to grow old with Tithonus – she had to greet the birth of each new day until the end of time.)

Napoleon, the Tithonus of St Helena! But what did Hudson Lowe turn him into? One of the giant tortoises that live to a great age and roam the gardens of Plantation House? How ironic if it was the one that fell over a cliff in 1918, broke its shell and died.

The only records of Napoleon's medical history that may be considered acceptable are those of the four doctors who actually looked after him (the Establishment's going to love that!). Although their value may have been challenged on a number of counts, these individual records *as they left the pen* nevertheless remain the essential starting point of any account of Napoleon's exile. Unfortunately, they do not appear to have been as diligently studied as they might have been by those, including doctors (maybe especially doctors?), striving for the truth – but what is truth? How will we even know when it's within our grasp? Alas, we have to face facts: the truth about the past is unattainable; the most we can hope for is *informed* opinion, and even that can be manipulated to suit vested interests of one kind or another.

* * *

If any sense is to made of the Emperor's exile on St Helena, two questions need to be answered. The first, "Why did his medical management fall apart at the seams so disastrously?" has never been addressed, let alone answered. The second, "What was the cause of his death?" needs to be broken down into two parts: "What actually killed him?" and "What else was he suffering from at the time?"

And now, *mon ami(e)*, come with me while I lead you by the hand to the answers to these two questions.

~2~
Escape from France...

(JUNE 20 – JULY 7, 1815)

To answer our first question, "Why did Napoleon's medical management fall apart at the seams so disastrously?", we have to go back to Laon where he came up against political reality. But why so far back? Because, as I said, Laon marked the first in the chain of events that were beyond his control and finally delivered him into British hands – specifically, and this proved of critical importance, the hands of the Royal Navy.

Napoleon had convinced himself that he should stay in Laon to organize the defence of Paris. He knew he'd be more successful at keeping the Allies out of France than they would be at taking Paris. He also knew there was trouble brewing at home, but this he regarded as a minor inconvenience that would fade away when his armies were once again victorious (and he had once again established himself as emperor/dictator). So, if he could get Soult's army to join with Grouchy's at Laon, and then bring the armies of the Rhine and the Jura, both under highly competent generals, into the attack against the Allied east flank, he would make Wellington's victory look rather less of an English hooley. But was he paying sufficient attention to the quality of his commanders – his original poor choices of Soult and Grouchy? Could he rely on them to show initiative and common-sense at the second time of asking? Had they been Suchet, Davout or Murat . . .? Ah! that would have been a different kettle of fish entirely and he would scarcely have been in his present predicament.

Napoleon's planning was, however, brought to a juddering halt when he was confronted by his Secretary of State: Hugues Maret, Duke of Bassano, a diplomat of no mean achievement. He knew precisely what was happening in Paris, and had the best interests of both Napoleon and France at heart – regrettably, not one and the same at this moment. Nevertheless, Maret was equal to the occasion and talked to his Emperor like a Dutch uncle, eventually impressing on him that if he didn't show himself in Paris and calm the situation the Assembly might well surrender behind his back, and that would well and truly leave him up the creek without a paddle.

But still confident that he held the trump cards, Napoleon set off for Paris, vowing to return in five or six days' time. He rode hard through the night and at about 8am a rather crumpled emperor slid from his horse at the gates of the Elysée Palace.

Before doing anything else he had a hot bath, a much-needed snooze and something to eat. The pleas of his cabinet ministers to dissolve the Assembly without delay could wait until he was refreshed and ready in his own time to get down to business.

And how, do I hear you ask, was it that Napoleon, apparently secure among his apparently loyal people in the middle of Paris, was to find himself at sea in the Atlantic Ocean, a sitting duck for the Royal Navy? The two chief players in the answer are Public Opinion (otherwise power to the people) and Field Marshal Gebhard Leberecht von Blücher, Prince of Wahlstadt, the seventy-three-year-old Commander-in-Chief of the Prussian army, who was still at war and marching on Paris. One after the other they made it perfectly plain to Napoleon that his world had changed.

For the next three or four days messages sped back and forth between the Chamber of Deputies and Napoleon and his ministers. The main negotiator in the Chamber was its President, Joseph Fouché. Now, if you want an example of downright treachery, look no further than Joseph Fouché; a supercilious bastard who believed the sun shone out of his fundament! He had been appointed, reluctantly, by Napoleon as his Minister of Police. He was also in not very secret correspondence with Wellington; Francis, Emperor of Austria; Louis XVIII and doubtless many others telling them all about Napoleon's intentions; however, he made sure that he also acquired a working knowledge of the Allies' intentions – and not for Napoleon's benefit either.

Napoleon continued on blithely arguing that if the nation rose as one, the enemy could be overcome, but if the Chambers frittered the time away all would be lost. To this end, he told them, through his ministers, they should invest him with the extraordinary power of temporary dictatorship (except that if he had anything to do with it there would be nothing temporary about it). But Fouché soon put a stop to this bit of nonsense with a resolution to the effect that any attempt to dissolve the chamber would be regarded as treason and any person who tried to do so would be considered a traitor.

The debate in the Chamber of Deputies went on at bad-tempered length until one member thankfully had a flash of clear-sightedness: "Separate the cause of Napoleon from that of the nation," his voice rang out in the inspirational wilderness. "One individual only stands between us and peace!" The Chamber fell silent. Until Napoleon was removed from the equation there really was no hope of peace for France.

So, Napoleon must abdicate if any progress were to be made. In their first flush of enthusiasm that the end was in sight the Deputies proposed to let him abdicate in favour of his son, Napoleon, King of Rome. And much good would that do anybody as the King was a virtual captive at his grandfather's court in Vienna. Power in France would land up once again in the hands of the Bourbons, "Long live Louis XVIII!"

Napoleon began to wonder whether he should abdicate at all. But when, after a night's sleep, the Deputies actually voted for abdication, he saw clearly that if he didn't go voluntarily, he would be removed forcibly and that would mean goodbye to any thought of Napoleon II. He abdicated. The Assembly duly proclaimed Napoleon II to be the Emperor of France.

The next step was to get Napoleon I out of Paris and on his way out of the country. To help plant the boot in the best place in his anatomy, the Provisional Government asked the Allies to grant passports and assurances of safe passage to allow him and his family to travel to the United States of America. Blücher would have nothing to do with the idea and Wellington said he had no authority from his Government. (But anyway this was just one of Fouché's ruses to let the Allies know what Napoleon's next move was likely to be.) So, while waiting for the necessary paperwork, Napoleon retired to Malmaison, Josephine's old home on the banks of the Seine some eight miles from the centre of Paris.

We are now at June 25 and Blücher had reached the northern outskirts of Paris. Davout, Napoleon's Minister of War, knew that once Blücher discovered where his quarry was to be found, he *would* be found and executed on the spot – Davout was in no doubt about that. If you were a Prussian wouldn't you want to exact retribution for the appalling cruelty dispensed by the French during their withdrawal through your country in 1813?

When all this was explained to him, Napoleon reacted in a manner that might be expected of a lesser mortal: seeing what he believed to be a way of exploiting the situation to his advantage, he first offered to advise on the defence of Paris and when this was rejected out of hand, he then offered his services to the Government in the rank of general, nothing more exalted, and lead the army against the enemy. This also was treated with the contempt it deserved.

Didn't he understand that if his offer was accepted, not only would it put paid to any hope of a peace settlement with the Allies, it would also stir up trouble throughout the country? The Government had had enough; Napoleon was given his marching orders and told to leave the country whether he had passports and safe conducts or not. (Throughout all these negotiations, Fouché and Provisional Government may, for all practical purposes, be regarded as one and the same.)

Preparations for departure were proceeding at an unhurried pace until Blücher discovered where Napoleon was staying and despatched the 8th Hussars and two battalions of infantry to take the bridge at Chatou, half-a-mile or so lower down the river but leading directly to Malmaison. The Prussians arrived to find the bridge destroyed – the loyal (to Napoleon) Davout had acted in time.

Sizeable quantities of the imperial silver, dinner services, linen of every description, in fact everything, so it seemed, that would enable the imperial exiles to live in their customary style, was piled into a couple of waiting coaches under the guiding hand of Napoleon's head valet, Louis Marchand. Considering that instructions had been issued (by Fouché) about the quantities to be taken, the guards must have nodded (or taken backhanders) when the imperial servants removed this plunder from the royal palaces. Marchand's own coach had already been filled with his master's personal effects, and books had been collected from the libraries. Tearful goodbyes were stammered. Marie Waleska, with their son, came to perform symbolic suttee by begging to accompany Napoleon wherever he might go, but she was refused. His step-daughter, Hortense, Josephine's daughter by Alexandre Beauharnais, was, not unsurprisingly, there to say farewell – she gave him a belt stitched full of diamonds to see him through hard times.. Did any of those gathered on that day even guess that they would never see their beloved Emperor again? No one yet guessed what was in store for him.

At about 5pm on June 29 Napoleon Bonaparte stepped into his coach and took his leave of Paris, bound for the port of Rochefort on the Biscay coast. He may well have thought his escape to be in his own hands, but he couldn't have been more wrong.

Fouché wanted him out of the country with all haste to pacify the Allies and ensure that the peace negotiations would run smoothly to their conclusion. He had taken steps to ensure that the journey to the coast would suffer a minimum of hiccups, and had even arranged that when Napoleon arrived at Rochefort, he would find two frigates, *La Salle* and *La Méduse*, anchored off the Ile d'Aix, waiting to take him to America.

Unfortunately for Napoleon, by the time he reached Rochefort, the political situation in Paris had changed and it had now been decided that he should be kept in France until his fate was decided, rather than have him at large in the United States where heaven knew what devilment he might get up to. But if he did get to America the countries of Europe didn't want him back playing soldiers in their bailiwicks; let him have a go at recovering some of the erstwhile French possessions over there, if that would keep him happy. An at-large Bonaparte would be a bloody nuisance to all concerned. Fouché responded to the changed situation with characteristic deviousness: he didn't withdraw the frigates from their station, instead he instructed (by telegraph) the two captains not to sail until the passports had arrived – and we all know that was never going to happen.

Incidentally, the telegraph had been introduced in 1793, employing a form of semaphore. In *The Count of Monte Cristo* by Alexandre Dumas, it played a significant role in one of the count's acts of revenge. Alexandre Dumas was, by the bye, the illegitimate son of a marquis who had been a general in the armies of the Revolution. After the defeat at the battle of the Nile, the French generals lost confidence in Bonaparte and sent Dumas, a giant of a man in size, courage and reputation, to confront him with their demand that the Directory should recall the army. With a calculated display of icy anger, Bonaparte well and truly put Dumas in his place; the wretched man left without even saying why he had come. Napoleon had shown his generals who was master.

But the fugitives from Paris faced greater problems than Fouché had foreseen – the Royal Navy appeared on the scene. While England had been at war with France, a squadron of the Channel Fleet, commanded since 1810 by Admiral Lord Keith, had blockaded the Atlantic coast. With the war over, the blockade had been lifted, but when Napoleon, now the only problem, was known to be making for the Atlantic coast, Keith on his own initiative resumed the blockade. The squadron, under the command of Rear-Admiral Sir Henry Hotham, had an unenviable task as the nature of the coast with its estuaries and islands offered numerous channels of escape and Hotham had only a limited number of ships under his command. Fortunately, he was well served by his officers, particularly by the captain of the *Bellerophon*, a 74-gun warship. Captain Frederick Maitland had, like Hotham, a valuable knowledge of the area from wartime experience.

When news of Napoleon's progress towards Rochefort came through, Hotham's flagship the *Superb*, 74 guns, was on duty at Quiberon Bay. Hotham at once set sail south. Maitland, though, found himself at the sharp end and no mistake: if Napoleon escaped, he would be the one who carried the can. However, he was a first rate seaman and made use of all his experience to ensure that no vessel slipped past without being boarded and inspected.

* * *

And now, *mon ami(e)*, you understand that, after Waterloo, Napoleon thought he could still regroup his forces and save France. Unfortunately, he didn't realize that he was up against Public Opinion and the public had had enough. He abdicated and fled the country, avoiding capture by Blücher by a hair's breadth and reaching the coast just as the Assembly in Paris changed its mind and decided it would prefer to keep him in France, for the time being at any rate.

~3~
… *and into the arms of the Royal Navy*

(JULY 8 – 16, 1815)

A few days after his arrival at Rochefort Napoleon got out of bed for the last time on French soil. He had decided it would probably attract the least attention if he left from the seaside village of Fouras and that was where the boats from *La Salle* and *La Méduse* collected him and his entourage. On this same day, July 8, Louis XVIII had made his entry into Paris to the resounding cheers of his people (as that fickle lot now were).

Napoleon and his staff scratched their heads for ways of evading the blockade. The pity of the whole situation was that propositions with any practicality at all were most likely to fail; the airy-fairy ones, such as sailing in a Danish merchantman hidden in a brandy barrel, would land him in British hands as a prisoner with his imperial dignity in tatters.

In the hope of gathering some fresh ideas, Napoleon sent Las Cases and Savary under a flag of truce to the *Bellerophon*. Maitland received them with great courtesy and they were invited to a working breakfast. The ostensible purpose of their visit was to enquire about the passports, but in reality it was to see what information they could pick up about British intentions – not as daft as it might seem as Las Cases hid the fact that he spoke English fluently. With the British being deficient in French (now there's a surprise!), they would be quite likely to indulge in careless talk while working out how to express themselves in French. The ploy worked to the extent that Las Cases gathered the distinct impression that the ex-emperor would be favourably received in England if he surrendered voluntarily.

On Las Cases's subsequent visits his companions began paving the way for Napoleon to be taken to England. Maitland, however, had no authority to promise anything; he had been caught holding a very hot chestnut that lacked any precedent whatsoever; he was simply acting as his nature demanded of him. Nevertheless, he was doing his damnedest to get Napoleon to surrender to him, believing the Government would act honourably – he just didn't allow for the double-dealing of the politicians back home.

However, should Napoleon find himself in English hands, his future had already been planned in outline: at the end of June the British Government, in the persons of Lord Liverpool, the Prime Minister; Lord Castlereagh, the Foreign Secretary; and Lord Bathurst, the Colonial Secretary, had realized it was going to be them, the British Government, that would get landed with the problem of what to do about Napoleon (and doing it) when eventually he fell into the hands of one or other of the Allies. They thereupon decided that he would be regarded as a prisoner-of-war with the rank of general and would be treated as such. Where to imprison him was more of a headache. Apart from England, which didn't fill them with any great enthusiasm, a remote Scottish castle, Malta, St Helena, the Cape of Good Hope or any other colony, for heaven's sake, where they wouldn't lose too much sleep worrying about his security.

Maitland's background helped in a situation like this since, in addition to his naval training, he was a Scottish aristocrat – a grandson of the sixth earl of Lauderdale – and would instinctively have some idea of how to behave honourably, particularly when having to deal with a man, whether emperor or not, in Napoleon's predicament. On the other hand, the Government in England was concerned only with how best to deal with a thorny political problem that had tricky international ramifications. [Lord Keith happened to be another Scottish aristocrat – the Honourable George Elphinstone, youngest son of Lord Elphinstone. Sir Henry

Hotham was an English variation on the theme being the third son of the second Lord Hotham of South Dalton (in the East Riding of Yorkshire) – just thought you'd like to know].

The *Bellerophon*, incidentally, was the first ship of that name to be commissioned into the Royal Navy. She was named after one of the heroes of Greek mythology, though he achieved this eminence in a somewhat dubious manner. The son of Glaucus (whose ghost frightens horses to this day), he began life as Hipponous, but when he murdered Bellerus he took the name Bellerophon and fled to the court of the king of Tiryns. The king's wife did what mythological king's wives are prone to do and promptly fell for him. He spurned her advances and, as he should have anticipated, she told her husband that he had tried to seduce her. The king shrank from killing a guest and sent Bellerophon to his father-in-law, the king of Lycia, with a letter asking him to do the deed instead. He, too, was reluctant to kill a guest and instead imposed a variety of tasks on him, hoping to get out of his quandary at second-hand, as it were.

The first task was for Bellerophon to fight the Chimaera, a fire-breathing monster. Being the current owner of Pegasus, the winged horse, he was able to fly over the monster and either shoot it with his arrows or kill it by stuffing its flaming mouth with lead. (Mythology is worse than history for arriving at an agreed version of what they all got up to.) The king of Lycia next sent Bellerophon against the Amazons whom he defeated – heroes didn't count the odds. On his return he found himself ambushed by the king's guards and proceeded to slay the lot, thereby winning the king's admiration and his daughter's hand in marriage. If only the story could have ended there but alas, the end of the hero's life was not a happy one. Apparently, he got a bit above himself and, mounted on Pegasus, attempted to reach Mount Olympus – the home of the gods on the mountain of that name in Greece. An infuriated Zeus threw him from his horse and badly lamed him. Bellerophon ended his days in misery. Pegasus gained Olympus. That's mythology for you!

By this time Napoleon was getting distinctly worried. The possibility of escape was becoming fainter by the day and it would be a very bad idea to fall into the hands of the Bourbons, whether by capture or surrender, since they were liberally executing Bonapartists. Indeed, on the very day, July 15, that Napoleon went aboard the *Bellerophon*, an officer was despatched from Paris to the captain of *La Salle* ordering him to deliver Napoleon to the British for onward transmission to Paris. And even if he did make it to the United States of America there was a growing likelihood that he would be shipped back to England at the request of the Russians.

All in all, Napoleon decided that his best chance lay with Maitland. Negotiations for a possible surrender had gone well, so early in the morning of July 15 he boarded *L'Epervier*, a brig of war accompanying the frigates, and set out for the *Bellerophon*. While the brig was still some way off, Maitland ordered the ship's barge to meet it and take Napoleon on board. As the barge began its return journey, the brig's crew broke into the loudest cheering you would be likely to hear this side of Davy Jones's locker; "*Vive l'Empereur*" echoed across the sea until the Emperor disappeared from their sight for ever.

Maitland had sent the barge because the *Superb*, blessed with a favourable wind, was now close by and he wanted Napoleon up the gangway and all formalities completed before his commanding officer appeared on the scene. It was bad enough that he had received no instructions as to how Napoleon should be treated: as ex-emperor, as general officer, as prisoner-of-war. Maitland paled at the thought of Hotham appearing in the middle of it all with the formidable challenges of etiquette and protocol this would pose; he saw the barge as the solution. It worked. [Should you choose to believe that Maitland did all this so that he would go down in history as the man who captured Napoleon, that's up to you.]

General Bertrand, Napoleon's Grand Marshal, was first up the ship's side and confirmed for Maitland what he already knew – that

Napoleon was on the barge. Sure enough, the next minute Napoleon appeared, outfitted in the uniform of a Chasseur à Cheval of the Imperial Guard, and made for the quarter deck where he removed his hat in salute and announced "Sir, I am come to throw myself on the protection of your Prince and laws" (in French, of course). Despite the Royal Marine guard of honour being drawn up on the break of the poop, arms were not presented. This was not an act of discourtesy, simply that ceremonial acts and displays were not indulged in before six o'clock in the morning! Maitland himself was courtesy personified.

He first ushered the ex-emperor into the great cabin where, at Napoleon's request, all the ship's officers were presented to him. Napoleon was next given a tour of the *Bellerophon*, all the while asking the most penetrating of questions as if on the morrow he would be taking her to sea. This over, they all sat down to an English breakfast. Napoleon ate little but questioned a lot, this time about the English way of life. Having placed himself under the captain's protection, he genuinely believed he would be granted sanctuary in England where he would end his days in deep retreat as a country gentleman under an assumed name. A pseudonymous Napoleon! Some hope, even if this miracle had come to pass.

Meanwhile Napoleon's compatriots had come aboard from *La Méduse* and were allocated their cabins for the voyage, the ladies and senior members of Napoleon's suite getting those of the *Bellerophon's* officers – whose views on the matter were neither here nor there. Most of the rest of the day was spent transhipping Napoleon's baggage, his personal belongings being taken to the captain's cabin which was to be his throughout the voyage. By early afternoon the *Superb* had laid to and Maitland was taken across to report to Admiral Hotham who was delighted. Napoleon had been taken unconditionally – that was how the Government would wish it.

On his return to the *Bellerophon*, Maitland told Napoleon that Hotham would visit him later in the day. As if to demonstrate what it was all about on his side, Napoleon sent his Grand Marshal, accompanied by Maitland, over to the *Superb* to ensure that Hotham was alert to the protocol required when meeting the Emperor. Hotham followed his instructions to the letter and once they had all got to know each other, Napoleon played host at a dinner prepared by his servants (Maitland had profited from the experience of the English breakfast) and eaten off the imperial dinner service. The Admiral was seated on his right and the Countess Bertrand on his left at what was just the start of an evening of great bonhomie. It ended with Hotham inviting the Emperor to join him for breakfast.

Next morning, the crew of the *Bellerophon* made up for their ceremonial deficiencies the previous day. Arms were presented, yards were manned and every opportunity taken to welcome and honour the Emperor. For his part, Napoleon indulged in what he was good at: after the Royal Marine guard of honour had presented arms they were reviewed and complimented on their turnout. On his arrival on board the *Superb*, which also had its crew strung out in salute along the yards, he continued reviewing and complimenting anything that stood still for long enough. Breakfast was another English affair and he didn't eat much, but this did nothing to still his endless questioning or dampen his enjoyment. The camaraderie continued till noon when the Emperor was returned to the *Bellerophon*. It was like coming home from a day at the races!

That afternoon, with the Emperor Napoleon aboard, the *Bellerophon*, accompanied by two smaller vessels, set sail for England. The Emperor Napoleon had no idea what lay in store for him.

* * *

And now, *mon ami(e)*, you will understand how it was that Napoleon fell into the arms of the Royal Navy rather than those of an army unit as might have been expected. This had a truly profound influence on the future course of his health.

~4~
Napoleon's surgeon, RN

(JULY 16 – AUGUST 7, 1815)

In the short term Napoleon could consider himself fortunate to be under the protection of Captain Maitland. He was emperor for ten more days, behaving and being treated as such. He had escaped the Prussians, who would undoubtedly have executed him on the spot, and in the flight to Rochefort he had evaded the manoeuvres of Louis XVIII's Government to bring him back to Paris where, again, execution would have been his almost certain fate. It didn't bear thinking about! As far as he was concerned he was on his way to England where he would enjoy a comfortable retirement as a wealthy foreign gentleman. He was aware that he would be sent to a remote part of the countryside, but he knew that given time he would be able to charm his way into society even if the Government was hell bent on his security. He was quite looking forward to the challenge!

He and Maitland got on extremely well during the voyage from Rochefort to Tor Bay – and by no means entirely because Maitland bent over backwards to ensure that imperial protocol was preserved at all times by all on board. Among the officers presented to the Emperor when he came aboard the *Bellerophon* had been the ship's surgeon, Mr Barry O'Meara (pronounced O'Mara – he was Irish). The Emperor's subsequent tour of the ship ended on the poop deck where it had started. O'Meara was still there.

"Are you the *chirurgien major*?" Napoleon asked.

"Yes, I am," O'Meara answered in fluent Italian to Napoleon's considerable relief. Here was someone he could talk to, rather than indulging in stilted question and answer moments.

"And what is your native country?"

"Ireland."

"Where did you study your profession?"

"In Dublin and London."

"Which of the two is the better school of physic?"

"I think Dublin is better for anatomy, and London for surgery."

"Oh," he said with a smile, "you say Dublin because you are an Irishman."

O'Meara begged his pardon. "I said so because it is true. In Dublin the subjects for dissection are procured at a fourth the price paid for them in London and the professors are equally good."

Napoleon then asked what actions he had seen and where he had served. Amongst the places was Egypt, whereupon Napoleon pricked up his ears. He was still obsessed with the Orient, though maybe not so magnificently as when he had pictured himself a born-again Alexander of Macedon. The consequence of this, his expedition to Egypt, may have been a cultural success but in the end it was a military disaster. His attempt to out-Alexander Alexander and conquer the world by marching through Syria and striking a blow against England by colonizing India (the other version is that his intention had been to take his army from one end of the Ottoman Empire to the other and on through the Balkans back to France) got him all of one hundred and twenty-five hard miles into hostile territory before he had to turn back, having achieved nothing except a casualty list approaching a third of the total force (five hundred killed in action, seven hundred dead from the plague, two thousand five hundred wounded). Nevertheless, when he deserted his army and returned to France, he did so, in his own eyes, as a victorious hero. He had been appointed Commander-in-Chief of the Army of the Orient by the Directorate, largely to get him out of their hair; six months after his return he had been voted First Consul! The man had certainly got something.

Incidentally, the British officer who negotiated the surrender of the abandoned French army was the Admiral in command of the Mediterranean Fleet, a certain Lord Keith. He behaved like the gentleman he was and allowed the troops to return to France with all the honours of war – they could leave with their arms and flags and not have to surrender them as trophies.

But to return to the poop deck of HMS *Bellerophon*: This explains why Napoleon was tickled pink when O'Meara mentioned that he had once messed in a house that had previously been used as stables for his horses – British officers living in accommodation fit only for the horses of General Bonaparte! *Mais certainement*!

Since exercise was of first importance to his existence, Napoleon could usually be found pacing up and down the deck talking to whoever could understand him. He always had a word with O'Meara and would ask him to come to his rescue by translating or explaining something. Then one morning he asked him to treat an orderly officer who had been taken seriously ill: his personal physician, M. Maingaud, was vomiting his heart out in his cabin – seasickness is no respecter of the medical profession. But even when Maingaud had found his sea legs, O'Meara continued to care for the officer; a consequence, no doubt, of the answers he gave to Napoleon's searching questions about the nature and progress of the illness – Napoleon was no slouch when it came to an understanding of medicine.

The *Bellerophon* rounded Berry Head on July 24 and dropped anchor a half-mile off Brixham Quay. An officer was landed with dispatches for London. General Bonaparte, now officially in the custody of the British Government, was safely on board a British warship in British waters. On his staff was a French doctor prepared to accompany him into exile. So far so good.

Bellerophon's officer duly returned from London with dispatches ordering Maitland to up anchor and sail for Plymouth on what turned out to be the start of a ten-day summer cruise off the south Devon coast courtesy of HM Government.

Soon after their arrival in Plymouth on July 31, they were visited by Major-General Sir Henry Bunbury, Under Secretary of State, bearing the glad tidings that St Helena, not the leafy groves of England, was to be General Bonaparte's next home. This was the outside of enough for M. Maingaud who lost no time in letting Bertrand know that the salons of fashionable Parisian society had more to offer a rising star of the medical profession than exile on a remote island in the south Atlantic. *Pas problème.* Napoleon was still on board the *Bellerophon* and O'Meara was the ship's surgeon. Anyway, Maingaud had only been a locum for Dr Fourreau de Beauregard, Napoleon's doctor on Elba, who had been unable to get to Rochefort in time – he was in Paris being elected to the Chamber of Representatives. He would turn up in due course.

Meantime, both Maitland and Hotham got right royal epistolical rollockings from Lord Keith. It appeared that the First Lord of the Admiralty, Lord Melville, had interviewed the *Bellerophon's* officer and been told how General Bonaparte had been treated with imperial respect when on board the two battleships. Melville was seriously uptight that if this continued, Napoleon would use it to his advantage and cast a spell on his guardians – as indeed had happened when he took the title of King of Elba. He at once wrote to Keith with orders that Napoleon was henceforward to be regarded as a general officer with the privileges appropriate only to that rank; he was also a prisoner-of-war! When this bombshell was communicated to the General, it upset his composure and no mistake!

He had put himself under the protection of Captain Maitland (who although lacking the authority to promise anything, did, nevertheless, sincerely believe that his promises would be honoured by the British Government); he had *not* surrendered and anyway England was not at war with the legitimate government of Louis

XVIII. But his protestations achieved nothing and the status of prisoner-of-war festered away at the top of his list of grievances for virtually the rest of his life. The Government (i.e. the three ministers) reckoned that this status allowed them to act as they wished. The other Allies had approved the British behaviour at the Convention of Paris and were not exactly reluctant to have the problem taken out of their hands. Consequently the Government was able to persuade Parliament to lend the whole unsavoury business a veneer of respectability with an Act of Indemnity – which meant they could continue to do as they wished with no fear of a legal comeback.

However, a new problem arose in Plymouth in the shape of the local population. No matter their opinion of Napoleon, he was the greatest event to strike Plymouth since Drake and his game of bowls – this may well have been apocryphal but the arrival of 'Boney' in their harbour certainly was not. An almost continuous flotilla of boats encircled the *Bellerophon*, with local traders attempting to flog their wares to the sailors and adopting all manner of tricks to make contact. The sailors, for their part, held up bulletin boards announcing what Napoleon was doing at that particular moment. Every time he appeared on deck, the crowds on the dockside burst into enthusiastic cheering and Napoleon milked the situation for all he was worth.

Under orders to prevent any contact between his sailors and the local citizenry, Maitland knew this state of affairs could not be allowed to continue. He also had the added worry that Napoleon's supporters who were determined to get him onto dry land had, by devious means, concocted the trial of a British admiral on the completely false charge of dereliction of duty and had obtained a writ of habeas corpus. So, when the trial took place Napoleon would be compelled to appear as a witness – and who knew where that might lead? On top of it all Maitland was waiting until the ship booked to take General Bonaparte to St Helena put in an appearance and any idiot could see that a ship-to-ship transfer in Plymouth harbour would simply be asking for trouble. The obvious solution was to arrange a rendezvous off a less Bonapartist stretch of coast. Captain Maitland was therefore instructed to extend the cruise round Start Point and on if needs be.

Fourreau de Beauregard had still not turned up. Bertrand now really did have *un problème* which needed something done about it, and that something was O'Meara. Napoleon liked him, the two got on well together and he was professionally more than acceptable. In his role of Grand Marshal, Bertrand first sounded out Napoleon who gave his agreement in principle. He then got General René Savary, Duke of Rovigo, to see what his new friend O'Meara thought of the idea, particularly in view of the destination. If he was in favour, Bertrand would send him a confirmatory letter. O'Meara was perfectly happy to go ahead so long as the British Government and Captain Maitland were of the same mind and so long as his stipulations were acceptable. [I think you should take note of the fact that O'Meara linked his commanding officer on equal terms with the government. The Royal Navy was quite clear that its officers were responsible to their commanding officer, whether he was the captain of their ship or an admiral in command of their station, and to no other – after all, the Royal Navy *is* the Senior Service. This protocol was one of the sources of the later troubles on St Helena.]

Maitland recommended acceptance, again with the proviso that the British Government and, this time *his* senior officer, Lord Keith gave it their blessing. All this took place on the third of August, the day before the *Bellerophon* left Plymouth. At the rendezvous, which turned out to be off Dartmouth, Bertrand officially laid the proposal before Maitland and O'Meara. It was immediately communicated to Lord Keith who summoned O'Meara to come aboard his flagship the *Tonnant*, an 80-gun warship captured from the French by Nelson at the battle of the

Nile and commissioned into the Royal Navy.

Incidentally, valuable information about a ship's capabilities was conveyed in the number of guns she carried. Thus the fact that Keith's *Tonnant* had 80 guns did not make her a 'better' ship than, say, the two-decker, 74-gun *Bellerophon*; in fact, she didn't sail so well as she was longer and less well proportioned and, moreover, was prone to hogging, which meant that the keel would gradually bend causing the bow and stern to sag. The two-decker 74s were better proportioned than the three-decker 74s and consequently sailed better; small wonder they were reckoned the most successful fighting ships in the age of sail. As beautiful at peace as they were deadly in battle.

Both *Bellerophon* and *Tonnant* were third raters which might suggest that they were not up to much, but assigning rates to fighting ships was simply a means of classifying them according to the number of guns they carried – it makes sense when you realize that each rate covered a range of numbers: first rate, 100 + guns; second rate, 84 –100 guns; third rate, 70 – 84 guns; and so on to sixth rate. (These numbers are the original 1751 numbers; most were raised by about ten in 1810.) Only the first three raters were reckoned fit for the line of battle.

O'Meara began by explaining to Lord Keith why he felt his stipulations – which he subsequently committed to paper and sent to Keith – were essential if he was to protect his own best interests. He was nobody's fool and could see the potential for trouble if he was to be serving two masters. By setting these conditions down in writing, he put on record that he remained an officer in the Royal Navy (and as such responsible to his commanding officer):

> MY LORD, – Application having been made to me yesterday by Count Bertrand, to accompany General Napoleon Bonaparte to St. Helena, in quality of surgeon (as the surgeon who embarked with him in France, is unwilling to proceed further); I beg to inform your

> lordship, that I am willing to accept that situation (provided it meets with your lordship's approbation), and also on the following conditions, viz. that it should be permitted me to resign the above situation, should I find it not consonant with my wishes, on giving due notice of my intention thereof. That such time as I shall serve in that situation, shall be allowed to count as so much time served on full pay in his majesty's navy, or that I shall be indemnified in some way for such loss of time as surgeon on full pay, as it may occasion to me. That I am not to be considered in any wise depending upon, or to be subservient to, or *paid* by the aforesaid Napoleon Bonaparte; but as a *British officer* employed by the British government; and lastly, that I may be informed, as soon as circumstances will admit, of what salary I am to have, and in what manner and from whom I am to receive it.

That should cover everything, you might think, but O'Meara really couldn't have been expected to allow for the completely bizarre. And a fat lot of good his stipulations did him anyway when push came to shove on St Helena.

Lord Keith was delighted beyond measure. Bertrand had taken a nasty problem out of his and the Government's hands and had come up with the perfect solution. It was imperative that, wherever he was going, General Bonaparte should be attended by a doctor. However, under the circumstances Keith had been wondering whether it might prove necessary to get him out of the way as quickly as possible, relying on naval surgeons until a permanent doctor was appointed. But could he do that with St Helena the destination? It would never do for the Government to let him sail, personally unattended, to an island with such an unhealthy reputation – vehemently denied, of course!

He told O'Meara that he couldn't order him to accept as it was such an extraordinary business without precedent in the naval service, but he advised him in the strongest terms to take the job.

(He wasn't going to let this answer to a maiden's prayer slip through his fingers.) The Government would feel obliged to him, he said, as they were most anxious that the General should be accompanied by a surgeon of his own choosing. He needn't worry that acceptance might have an adverse effect on his career since the position was perfectly consistent with his honour, and with the duty he owed to country and sovereign.

For his part the 29-year-old O'Meara was pleased that everything was going ahead – and with the approval of two such distinguished officers as Lord Keith and Captain Maitland. It was the determining moment in his life!

(By the bye, Fourreau de Beauregard never did turn up. When told where he would be going he, like Maingaud, decided he would be better off in Paris.)

And so, on August 7 the final preparations were in hand to send Napoleon on his way. All that remained was his transfer to HMS *Northumberland*, 74 guns, commanded by Captain Charles Ross and flying the flag of Rear-Admiral Sir George Cockburn. With his letter delivered to Lord Keith and Napoleon safely on board the *Northumberland*, O'Meara bade goodbye to Captain Maitland and was rowed across to take up his new appointment. (That he was still officially regarded as an officer in the Royal Navy is confirmed by his being listed in the Admiralty Muster Rolls as supernumerary surgeon on the *Northumberland*.)

Here, we too say goodbye to Captain Maitland, but before leaving him, I should like to quote the testimonial he had written for O'Meara a year earlier. It was dated November 5, 1814, and addressed to Dr Harness of the Transport Board:

> The attention and meritorious conduct of Mr Barry O'Meara while surgeon with me in the Goliath, calls upon me as an act of justice to him and of benefit to the service, to state, that during the fifteen years I have commanded some one of his majesty's ships, I

have never had the pleasure of sailing with an officer in his situation who so fully answered my expectations. Not being a judge of his professional abilities, though I have every reason to believe them of the first class, and know that to be the opinion of some of the oldest and most respectable surgeons in the navy, I shall only state, that during a period of very bad weather, which occasioned the Goliath to be extremely sickly, his attention and tenderness to the men was such as to call forth my warmest approbation, and the grateful affection of both officers and men. Were it probable that I should soon obtain another appointment, I know of no man in the service I should wish to have as surgeon so much as Mr.O'Meara. As, however, in the present state of the war that is not likely, I trust you will do me the favour of giving him an appointment, as encouragement to young men of his description, and believe me,

Dear Sir, &c. &c. &c.

FREDERICK L. MAITLAND

However, the state of the war did change when Napoleon escaped from Elba and O'Meara found himself posted to Plymouth as ship's surgeon on the *Bellerophon* under the command of Captain Maitland.

* * *

And now, *mon ami*(*e*), you will understand how it was that Napoleon landed up with a serving officer in the Royal Navy as his personal doctor on St Helena.

~5~
The General's health

(AUGUST 7 – OCTOBER 17)

HMS *Northumberland* had not been specially commissioned to take General Bonaparte to St Helena, she just happened to be in the right place at the right time. Admiral Sir George Cockburn, whose flag she was flying, was sailing to take up his appointment as Commander-in-Chief of the St Helena and Cape of Good Hope Naval Station. He was thus the perfect person to take responsibility for the General until the appointed governor arrived on the island.

Napoleon was permitted to take with him a limited number only of his household. Those selected were: his Grand Marshal, Count Henri Bertrand with his wife, Fanny, and their three children; Count Charles Montholon with his wife, Albine, and child; Count Emanuel Las Cases with his fifteen-year-old son, also Emanuel; Baron Gaspard Gourgaud, Master of the Horse; Louis Marchand, first valet; Cipriani, maitre d'hôtel; plus ten assorted domestics (six were Bertrand's), one of whom took his wife.

Accompanying the *Northumberland* were two troopships carrying the 53rd Regiment of Foot under the command of Brigadier-General Sir George Bingham and a company of Royal Artillery – someone had certainly got the wind up that there would be a concerted effort to free General Bonaparte. The surgeon with the Royal Artillery was one James Verling who you shall meet again in three years' time. Making up the convoy were the escorting sloops and frigates and a store ship.

Sir George Cockburn was heading towards a delicately

balanced diplomatic situation and he would have to tread carefully. The Honourable East India Company were Lords Proprietors of St Helena with all the rights of sovereignty and as such *they*, and not the British Government, had appointed the governor ever since 1673; the present holder of the office was Colonel Mark Wilks. This presented the British Government, in the person of Lord Henry Bathurst, Secretary of State for the Colonies, with an exercise in diplomacy. He was obsessive about the maintenance of security on the island and had no wish to run the slightest risk of antagonizing either the Company or the islanders who might respond by conspiring to gain Napoleon his freedom.

Accordingly, the Government got the Directors of the Company in London on side to the extent that the Directors gave Wilks and other members of the island's Council strict instructions on dealing with the situation, in particular how the governance of the island should be handled: Wilks was to remain governor while Sir George was to be in charge of all matters concerning Napoleon. Nevertheless, Wilks was ordered to execute any measures Sir George might feel necessary for ensuring Napoleon's security. Neither man was to be subordinate to the other. A recipe for disaster, you might think, but in the event it worked well as both men were sane and level-headed and had the same objectives: not only the security of Napoleon but also the furtherance of their own careers by creating favourable impressions back home in London. This they certainly succeeded in doing. Sir George rose to become Admiral of the Fleet; and Mark Wilks returned to his academic life well compensated for a job everyone acknowledged he had been doing outstandingly well.

The reason for all this pussyfooting around was on the high seas, thoroughly bored and behaving in a most boorish fashion. It was beginning to sink in that he was no longer emperor, all the privileges were gone and he could no longer impose his authority. His life would never be the same again – and that you may be sure about!

As the voyage progressed Cockburn became anxious about Napoleon's dietary habits; besides bolting his food, he was eating badly, never touching vegetables and preferring his meat highly seasoned; he was also drinking too much. Cockburn was afraid that, taken with his lack of proper exercise, he might not be in the best of condition by the time they reached St Helena. He suspected that Napoleon could be in danger of getting scurvy, a disease he was all too familiar with.

The *Northumberland* dropped anchor in the Jamestown roads on October 15 to a welcoming salute in honour of the new Commander-in-Chief of the Naval Station. The *Northumberland* responded. General Bonaparte received not so much as a misfire. (The commanding officer of the fort hadn't a clue whether the General should be saluted or not, and if so how many guns the salute should be.)

Now, as Napoleon is not to disembark for another two days it might be a good idea to assess his state of health at the start of his captivity on this reputedly unhealthy tropical island.

* * *

In the spring of 1815 Napoleon was perfectly fit and healthy. But he was forty-five and growing older does bring its penalties. He was doing well though, if his truly magnificent display of mental and physical energy in the fifteen weeks leading up to Waterloo is anything to go by: he rebuilt his Grande Armée, recruited vast numbers of extra workmen in the manufacturing of arms and munitions, re-modelled the civil and military administrations, introduced new laws and bye-laws, and restored his old empire with himself back on the throne.

Admittedly though, his physical condition was not what it once had been since he had put on a considerable amount of weight during his year on Elba. Maitland's impression was that of a remarkably strong, well-built man who had grown corpulent – but he had good teeth. Yes, he did appear corpulent, but the picture painted from life on the deck of the *Bellerophon* in Plymouth Sound shows also that his posture was bad and not helped by his choice of clothing. He needed a drill sergeant to order him to stand up straight, pull his stomach in and his shoulders back – and to change his couturier.

His behaviour at the start of the battle of Waterloo should dispel any suspicion that he was unfit. He spent the afternoon of the seventeenth of June giving chase with his cavalry in a torrential downpour. In the early evening, in a renewed downpour, he reconnoitred the entire Allied position on foot before returning to his headquarters at Le Caillou for a quick nap. Then on the day of the battle he was up at 1am to make a full inspection of his own outpost line before first light.

And no, he hadn't got piles and no, he didn't suffer from epilepsy.

* * *

When the *Northumberland* dropped anchor, Admiral Cockburn wasted no time. He immediately went ashore and, negotiating his way through a great congregation of curious islanders both black and white, reached the Castle, the governor's official residence. After a while he and Wilks emerged to be rowed out to the *Northumberland.* And then, once again, the uncertainty about Napoleon's place in the order of things showed itself. Instead of the Governor receiving a distinguished prisoner to his island, the Governor was presented to the ex-emperor. Oh dear! What would Lord Bathurst have to say if he ever found out?

With that formality out of the way, Cockburn and Wilks returned to the Castle to discuss where General Bonaparte might find a suitable residence. Not the easiest of tasks as all the best properties on the island belonged to the East India Company and were occupied – and no one was prepared to get out for a prisoner-of-State, as he now was. Eventually Governor Wilks suggested a place known as Longwood in the interior of the island and took Cockburn to have a look. Not wildly impressed, Cockburn nevertheless reckoned it would be worthwhile bringing the General to see it the next day.

But where was he to lodge until the chosen home was ready for occupation? Distinguished visitors were invariably invited to lodge at Plantation House, the governor's home, for the duration of their stay on the island. For whatever reason, this courtesy was not extended to the General. Consequently, Cockburn had to book him into a suitable lodging house. He selected one at the foot of the main street that was popular with travellers and generally accepted to be one of the best. This rat ridden, bug infested building belonged to Henry Porteous, superintendent of the East India Company's gardens. The fact that it was overrun with rats was of little concern; every other house on the island suffered the same inconvenience.

For the two days while Cockburn was ashore, General Bonaparte had nothing to do but contemplate the island where he might be compelled to end his days, though with a reasonable amount of luck his friends in Britain and Europe – and he still had influential friends – might secure his release. Unfortunately, his contemplations were not of the highest quality. Barry O'Meara may have said of Jamestown: "The first view of the town is pleasing, especially to those who have been long at sea, and resembles that of a scene at the theatre." The sight would, indeed, have been most pleasing to scorbutic sailors, since a stream ran down through the middle of the houses and its beds of watercress brought blessed relief from their scurvy.

Alas, O'Meara's first impressions didn't last long. "Nothing can be more desolate and repulsive" was his considered and heartfelt assessment. The island resembled nothing so much as a vast eruption of volcanic rock rejected by the Underworld, though one of the ladies of Napoleon's suite described it rather more picturesquely: "The devil must have shat the island as he flew from one world to the other," she is reputed to have said. (If anyone is taking bets on which lady was responsible, my money would go on Fanny Bertrand!)

Yet, despite his unfavourable contemplations Napoleon was only too happy to leave the *exécrable* ship behind. The sun had already set on the seventeenth when, accompanied by the Admiral and members of his suite including O'Meara, he landed at the Marino, a small street along the beach. Even at this late hour, soldiers with fixed bayonets had to force a way through the inevitable crowd to reach the main street and the Porteous lodging house. When it was too late to do anything about it, the Admiral realized that the curiosity of the islanders had turned the French arrivals into freaks on exhibition at a funfair. They made Napoleon's life a misery by hanging around the house desperate to catch a glimpse of their new resident – he couldn't come to the window of his room or walk down the stairs without being seen from outside. What made things worse was that they gawped in utter silence

Nevertheless, they may, perhaps, be forgiven. Their existence for hundreds of years had been devoted to producing the food to stay alive and to staving off the inevitable boredom in the best ways they could – riding, shooting, visiting, entertaining, private theatricals, race meetings. The arrival of ships in the harbour was always an occasion for jollity and civilized entertainment. Thus when, on October 11, HMS *Icarus* had sailed into Jamestown with the momentous news that the notorious Boney was soon to become one of them, the islanders' excitement knew no bounds. And when he actually stepped ashore, it was as if a play was being enacted in O'Meara's theatre.

The view from the anchorage, a night in a rat-infested boarding house, and the plague of citizens, aroused the General's suspicion that all might not be well for his future comfort.

* * *

And now, *mon ami(e),* you are informed about the health of General Bonaparte on his arrival at the island of St Helena. It was good, even if he was rather tubby, and perhaps harbouring a borderline deficiency of vitamin C.

~6~
Conditions of imprisonment

(OCTOBER 18, 1815 – APRIL 14, 1816)

Next morning, on the way to inspect the house at Longwood, Napoleon kept his eye open for somewhere decent to live. With him went the Admiral and Las Cases, his amanuensis. A mile-and-a-half out of town he caught a glimpse of a property he felt would be worth investigating on the way back but said nothing as he had been assured that Longwood was the most suitable residence on the island – after all it was the country seat of the lieutenant-governor.

Longwood had first come to notice some seventy years previously when the then governor carried out experiments in the cultivation of oats, wheat and barley. The initial results were promising enough to warrant the building of a barn. But the promise was not to be fulfilled and within three or four years the barn was converted into a house for the lieutenant-governor. Although based in London, the Directors of the East India Company were a well-informed lot and were not prepared to spend good money on the upkeep of an old barn.

As you might expect, Longwood was at first sight most unprepossessing (and at second and third if it comes to that). On all sides was a forest of gumwood trees, almost all the same size and, being nearly two thousand feet above sea level and exposed to a humid south-east trade wind, their bowed-down attitude reinforced the melancholy, brow-beaten appearance of the place. Their presence did nothing to shield the property from the eternal wind. The house itself had only five rooms, all ground floor, added on as required to meet the needs of whoever happened to be living there and with no heed given to order or convenience. It was in a shocking state of repair. Napoleon was, however, reassured that plans were already in hand for bringing the accommodation up to a standard adequate for himself and his staff – the Elysée Palace, perhaps?

He was welcomed by the Lieutenant-Governor, Lieutenant-Colonel John Skelton, Indian Army, and his wife Mary who spoke admirable French. Longwood had never been anyone's permanent home and Colonel Skelton made it plain that it was not his country residence from choice; like Napoleon, he had no option. Anyway he only lived there for three or four months in the year.

After inspecting the building, Napoleon was treated to a lunch that marked the start of a firm friendship.

As he was leaving, feeling more warmly disposed towards the world than he had for some time, he casually remarked that he would sooner make Longwood his home than stay in the town to be an object of curiosity. Little can he have realized just what he was saying!

On the return journey, at the remembered spot, he turned his little black horse, loaned by Governor Wilks, on to the track leading to The Briars, one of a half-dozen really pleasing estates on the island. The land was well cultivated; fruit and vegetables were plentiful and the water supply was good. One look was enough for Napoleon to tell the Admiral he would like to live there until the work at Longwood was completed – so long as the proprietor was happy with the arrangement. The current occupier was William Balcombe, Superintendent of Public Sales under the East India Company, who would become the purveyor to Longwood. He was happy.

A problem, though, was the accommodation: The house was small and Balcombe had a wife, two daughters, one of twelve and the other of fifteen, and two sons of around five or six. When Napoleon refused to be an inconvenience, a pavilion about thirty yards away from the main house came to the rescue. Here, Napoleon decided he would live with some of his staff and it was *they* who would just have to grin and bear the inconveniences of the arrangement – and they were many.

Cockburn also felt obliged to provide some sort of surveillance at The Briars and for starters he somehow or other managed to fit a captain of artillery with a sergeant and a few soldiers into the main house. Soon the pointlessness, not to mention the almost intolerable inconvenience of the soldiers' presence became apparent and they were removed.

Napoleon only once ventured outside the grounds He did, however, get much pleasure just wandering along the garden paths that took him into a confusion of orange trees, vines, roses, fuchsias and much else – mostly planted by previous residents.

On one occasion, when strolling with O'Meara, he stopped:

"Look," he said, gesturing at the breath-taking precipices all around, "look at your country's generosity! *This* is their magnanimity towards a wretched man who, in all good faith, put himself in their hands, mistakenly believing in what he imagined to be their national character. I once thought you were a free nation. I now see that your ministers laugh at your laws which are, like those of other nations, designed only to oppress the defenceless and shield the powerful, whenever your government has any object in view." *Plus ça change, plus c'est la même chose.*

With Napoleon their guest, the Balcombe family went out of their way to make life pleasant for him. They often invited him to the main house for a chat or a rubber of whist. And, to his delight, a firm friendship grew up with the two daughters, both proficient French speakers, in particular with Betsy, the younger.

While Napoleon was deriving such pleasure as he could at The Briars, Bertrand and Montholon, with their wives and children, and

Gourgaud and O'Meara continued to live at the Porteous lodging house where, thanks to Balcombe, they fed on the closest approach to home cooking he could provide. The only restrictions placed on the French at this time were that, if they went out, they should be accompanied by O'Meara or some other British officer or be followed by a soldier. Otherwise, they were at liberty to visit The Briars or wander wherever their fancy took them, forts and gun batteries excepted.

Insofar as the tedious monotony of life on St Helena permitted, every effort was made to make their existence tolerable – they were after all civilized human beings and a welcome addition to the social life of St Helena. They received calls from the Governor and Miss Laura Wilks (Mrs Wilks had left the island soon after Napoleon's arrival), from Colonel and Mrs Skelton, from members of the Council, from the officers of the military garrison and naval squadron and their wives and families and, as O'Meara so delightfully put it, from "most of the respectable families". Sir George gave several well-attended balls to which they were invited and to which, with the exception of Napoleon, they usually went. In their turn, they occasionally gave little evening parties.

Sir George devoted all his considerable energies to getting Longwood ready for Napoleon's occupation. He had no problem over carpenters and other specialist craftsmen as the *Northumberland* alone carried more than could be found on the entire island. He surprised the naturally bone-idle local workmen (mainly Chinese and some slaves) into an activity such as they had never witnessed on the island, let alone actually had to endure. He usually arrived shortly after sunrise and for almost two months Longwood resembled a scene in the dockyards when the fleet was fitting out for war. Every day two or three hundred seamen toiled up the steep side path, their heads and shoulders bowed under the timber and all the materials, even the stones, needed for the rebuilding; occasionally they were joined by fatigue parties from the 53rd

Regiment – thus drawing attention to the extent to which Napoleon and his welfare were the responsibility of the navy and Admiral Sir George Cockburn.

At last, Longwood House was ready to receive its new resident. The furniture, old-fashioned and of poor quality maybe, but the best that could be found, admittedly at horrendous expense, was in place. Yet, despite the refurbishment, the islanders were appalled that it had been selected as Napoleon's year-round home since it was generally regarded as the worst and most unpleasant spot on the island – and the locals should know.

Napoleon duly arrived at Longwood, escorted by Sir George, at four in the afternoon of December 10, 1815. His living quarters, in one wing of the building, consisted of a billiard room and drawing room, a small narrow writing room (later converted into a bedroom), a sort of antechamber in which a bath was put up, a dark low dining room, and the original bedroom.

The Montholons and their son had quarters in the opposite wing. Las Cases had a room in the middle of the house with his son sleeping in a cockloft reached through a hole cut in the ceiling of his father's room. The garrets were floored and turned into 'apartments' for Marchand, Cipriani and other members of staff; it was, however, impossible to stand upright except in their centres and at times they could become unbearably hot. O'Meara, Gourgaud and the current orderly officer lived in tents in the garden until extensions had been built for them. The Elysée Palace, anyone?

Because there was nothing suitable for them at Longwood, the Bertrands and their family lived at Hutt's Gate, about a mile away,. Although uncomfortable, it had been rented at their own request until the new house being built at Longwood was ready.

With everyone settling into a permanent routine, the time had come for Admiral Cockburn to attend to Napoleon's security. No longer would it be possible to continue with the lax arrangements of The Briars. The French had more opportunity to get up to mischief at Longwood and Cockburn had his instructions from London. So why, do I hear you ask, were they put in Longwood? Because they had to be somewhere where they could all be kept under surveillance together and where contact with the world outside could be strictly monitored. And about a mile away on the appropriately named Deadwood plain were encamped the 53rd Foot and the detachment of the Royal Artillery. All this was obviously going make General Bonaparte spitting mad, but Cockburn had his job to do.

He was, though, fully aware of the possible consequences should he overstep the mark:

"If I put sentinels in such a place, and insist on such and such measures, this man will shut himself up and never stir out. He will not live six months. I will not be the means of assassinating anybody." There spoke the prophet. "I will arrange matters so that he shall have liberty, and at the same time not afford him the least chance of escaping from the island, which is all that I can effect, or indeed care about."

Such, however, was the obsession of the Government with the General's security that Sir George had had his hands tied by London and was denied the freedom to act as he wished. In consequence, Napoleon was restricted to an area about twelve miles in circumference around the Longwood estate where he could ride or walk without being accompanied by a British officer. Nevertheless, the camp of the 2nd battalion of the 53rd Foot was inside this area and at Hutt's Gate, opposite the Bertrands, was an officer's guard. Visitors were allowed to enter the Longwood grounds if Bertrand had given them a pass. But this was no skin off the British nose as nobody could, in the first place, call on Bertrand without already being in possession of a pass from the Admiral, the Governor or Sir George Bingham, the Commanding Officer of the 53rd!

The orderly officer at Longwood was instructed to check the

physical presence of Napoleon twice in the twenty-four hours. This could be irritating in itself, but where the restrictions really started to make their presence felt was in the disposition of the guards. A subaltern's guard was posted at the entrance to Longwood at about six hundred paces from the house, and a cordon of sentries and pickets was posted round the twelve-mile limit. At nine o'clock in the evening the sentries closed in so that they were all in communication with one another, thus preventing anyone from entering or leaving the house without being seen and, if necessary, searched. Double sentries were posted at the entrance to Longwood which was constantly patrolled. After nine, Napoleon could not leave the house unless in the company of a field officer, and no one was allowed to pass through the cordon without the countersign. This went on till daylight.

Every landing place on the island, and indeed anywhere that could at the wildest stretch of the imagination be one, was picketed and sentries were stationed on every goat-path leading to the sea, even though virtually all the cliff paths would, in their own right, be insurmountable obstacles to the ungainly Napoleon.

The precautions to prevent his escape or rescue by sea were even more impressive. Ships could frequently be spotted from the island lookout posts as far as twenty-four leagues away, and always long before they could begin their approach to the shore. Two warships were on constant patrol round the island, one to windward and one to leeward, and they were signalled from the shore as soon as a ship was sighted. Every ship, except a British man-of-war, was escorted to the anchorage by one of these cruisers which stayed with her until she was either permitted to anchor or sent on her way. No foreign ships were allowed even to anchor unless they were in extreme distress, and in that case no one was permitted to land, while an officer from the escorting man-of-war was sent on board to take charge and ensure that no irregular communications were made.

Every fishing boat on the island was given a number and had to anchor at sunset under the supervision of a naval lieutenant. No boat, except the guard boats from naval vessels which were rowed round the island all night, was allowed to be at sea after sunset. Thus, short of actually incarcerating or enchaining him, Sir George took every possible precaution to prevent Napoleon's escape – or so we might think, until the next governor appeared on the scene.

The fears that Napoleon might escape were very real, and certainly the Government back in London was taking no chances – after all he *had* escaped from Elba, admittedly a different kettle of fish, and he *had* evaded the naval cordon. These restrictions added to the distress Napoleon undoubtedly felt in the unhealthy environment, both physical and mental, of Longwood. It would, indeed, be unwise to ignore the power of the emotions over bodily functions.

Many people were introduced to Napoleon in the early days at Longwood. They included the officers of the 53rd, the officers of the St Helena Regiments and their wives, and several of O'Meara's 'respectable' inhabitants. Some were invited to dine. Also officers and other 'respectable' passengers on ships outward bound from England or on their way home from India and China came to Longwood asking to be presented to the ex-emperor; they were refused only if Napoleon was indisposed or they had to leave the island before they could be fitted in. The respect shown him by his many English visitors could well have encouraged his hope that friends in England and a change in government might secure his release.

The boredom of his existence was partly attenuated by the great pleasure he took in reading, but even more he had this compulsive urge to record his version of events for posterity. But boring though life may have been, things were about to undergo an unwelcome change with the arrival, on April 14, 1816, of the frigate *Phaeton*, 38 guns, bearing the appointed governor, Lieutenant-

General Sir Hudson Lowe and Lady Lowe; Sir Thomas Reade, Deputy Adjutant-General; Major Gideon Gorrequer, aide-de-camp and Acting Military Secretary to Lowe; Mr Alexander Baxter, Deputy Inspector of Hospitals, and sundry other officers.

* * *

And now, *mon ami(e)*, you understand why the conditions of Napoleon's imprisonment during the first six months of his exile caused him considerable anguish which, in turn, could well be having an adverse effect on the function of his internal organs (you would know them as stress disorders).

~7~
Hudson Lowe – a suitable choice?

General Sir Hudson Lowe was in command of British troops in the south of France when he learned, on 1 August, 1815, of his appointment as Governor of St Helena. He was ordered back to London with all speed. On paper, his career indicated that he would be a suitable candidate for the job. At the age of forty-six, he was just a fortnight younger than the man he was to destroy. His father had been an impecunious army surgeon and consequently, when young Hudson joined the army he didn't enjoy the same social environment as his better-off colleagues. This, the powers-that-be reckoned, made him less likely to have the wool of Napoleon's charm pulled over his eyes. Furthermore, he made a habit of spending his leaves in either France or Italy, becoming fluent in the languages of both countries (and in Spanish as well).

His first posting after the outbreak of the Napoleonic Wars was to Ajaccio; when Corsica was abandoned he was sent to Elba and then to Minorca where he brought together a troop of Corsican *émigrés*, exiles and deserters and gave this unlikely bunch the title of Corsican Rangers. They turned up in Egypt and took part in the battle of Alexandria, but at the end of the campaign and with no more hostilities on the horizon he was put out to grass on half pay. Then in 1805 when Napoleon grew belligerent again, it was back to the Mediterranean with the rank of lieutenant-colonel to raise another band of Corsican Rangers to defend Sicily and pass the time blighting the trade of Murat's kingdom of Naples. This he was better able to do when, in 1806, the British captured Capri and he was given command of the island with a garrison composed of his Rangers, a regiment of Maltese soldiers and some British artillery. After a while Murat decided that something had to done about this British occupation – in the Bay of Naples! *Dieu m'en preserve!* – and in a carefully planned invasion forced Lowe to surrender. How could that be? Capri was an impregnable fortress and to surrender to an inferior force was unthinkable. Lowe's reputation in that part of the world sank like a lead balloon. But there was more to it than meets the eye. Lowe's cocked-up espionage activities on Capri point squarely in the direction of downright incompetence rather than contemptible military defeat.

When he was given command of the island, Lowe was also put in charge of espionage in the Mediterranean: he recruited a top class network centred on Naples. His courier was Antonio, a fisherman who came out from Naples at night under the pretext of fishing. Antonio and his sons were, in fact, the only loyal members of Lowe's organization.

The ring master of his network was Saliceti, the Minister of Police in Naples! He was a Corsican, a lawyer by profession and had been prominent in French politics during the Revolution. He was enjoying himself mightily as he had Lowe exactly where he wanted him. Every scrap of intelligence, both in and out, passed through his hands. He read every message sent by Lowe and if a reply was needed he would dictate a suitable one there and then. When he felt he couldn't answer directly, he played for time by arresting Antonio and his crew and imprisoning them for a few days. While they were locked up, his go-between with Lowe, by name Suzzarelli, demonstrated his talent for extracting money by asking for, and getting, the expenses necessary to save the poor wretches from being shot.

Antonio Suzzarelli was another Corsican who had once served as a British officer, maybe with the Corsican Rangers. He, too, had trained as a lawyer and was a man of many talents, some of which he was able to exercise while apparently serving Lowe. He was actually loyal for the first twenty days of his employment before being turned by Cipriani, the very same Cipriani who became Napoleon's maitre d'hôtel on St Helena. At this time Cipriani was known as Franceschi and was in Saliceti's confidential service – he was reputed to be the minister's natural son. Anyway, these two Corsicans, Suzzarelli and Cipriani, met in a taverna, swapped stories and emerged, both looking forward to implementing their family incomes. Suzzarelli, as Lowe's chief man in the field undertook all kinds of commissions for which he claimed expenses that would make a British politician blush. He also smuggled articles for Lowe often being paid in kind (plus expenses) which he subsequently sold in Naples at an absurd profit. He, too, enjoyed himself mightily.

One fine day Saliceti told Suzzarelli that he wanted to meet Lowe: "I should like to see this colonel of yours. A man may allow himself to be deceived for some months, but he who lets himself be humbugged so grossly for so many years must be a strange animal indeed!"

Suzzarelli set it all up and persuaded Lowe to come over to Naples and meet him at a small house on the beach. Saliceti, whose original intention had been to take Lowe prisoner, had decided against the plan – he couldn't imagine the British ever finding another commanding officer who would allow himself to be gulled so outrageously; he was too precious to lose. Alas, to the considerable disappointment of all involved, something persuaded Lowe to change his mind. (To give you an idea of just how gullible Lowe must have been, Suzzarelli later confessed that he had managed only once to deceive Saliceti, and that not completely.)

Members of Lowe's spy network were well paid by both sides and one apparently even ended up with a pension from the British Government! However, Lowe's method of paying them fairly takes the biscuit. They were paid in gold which Lowe, in his own house and with his own hands, had carefully baked inside loaves that resembled the bread the fishermen ate while fishing at night. He took this precaution in case his spies fell foul of the Neapolitan police spies – he hadn't a clue that his spies were their spies and that the loaves were taken straight to Saliceti!

But the best is yet to come: on one occasion in 1807 or 1808, Suzzarelli was sent to Vienna on a mission for Saliceti and thought it might be a bright idea if all expenses were paid by Lowe. When he told Lowe where he was going he mentioned that he would be able to gather information of the greatest value. Lowe fell for it. He not only gave Suzzarelli a generous sum for expenses, he also wrote a glowing letter of recommendation to the British ambassador in which he described Suzzarelli as a man in whom every confidence might be placed. And to make sure he got his money's worth, Lowe wrote to others of his acquaintance in the city who might be of help. And of help they were! Suzzarelli was well received by all, and thus did a veritable cornucopia of valuable intelligence find its way into French hands. His passport, issued by the ambassador when he left, styled him as *Il Signore Barone Suzzarelli*! And to round off the visit he obtained from the ambassador an order for payment of the salaries of the British agents on the continent! Quite an achievement!

By the end of 1808, King Joachim of Naples (Murat) had had enough of this carbuncle in the very bosom of Naples, he was seriously losing face. To the devil with Lowe's value to Saliceti! He would invade Capri and kick the invaders out.

To put Lowe off the scent, Suzzarelli persuaded him that an attack was being planned on the island of Ponza some sixty or so miles to the west (with a little bit of north in it) of Naples. Then, on the evening before the attack Suzzarelli sent Lowe a warning that it was actually Capri that was to be invaded the next morning. This served two purposes; one, that, whatever the outcome, Suzzarelli would not be compromised and, two, the short notice would put the wind up the garrison.

The Franco-Neapolitan invasion force consisted of between fifteen hundred and eighteen hundred men (including some elite troops), under the command of General Lamarque. It arrived, completely unopposed, under the rocky cliffs of Capri on October 5, supported by a naval force consisting of the frigate *Cerere*, the corvette *Renomée* and twenty-six gunboats. The British squadron, consisting of the frigate *Ambuscade*, 44 guns, three or four sloops and a flotilla of gunboats was nowhere to be seen. It had sailed away to the defence of Ponza!

Every known landing place on Capri was fortified. The town itself with the citadel and fort where Lowe and the rest of the garrison were to be found was reached by a narrow ascent of four or five hundred steps. Lowe had left this unfortified in the belief that heavy cannon could not be dragged up the side of a mountain. To prove him wrong, five hundred Frenchmen were harnessed to a couple of dozen four-pounder guns which, overnight, they hauled into place on Mount Solaro, overlooking the citadel. When they realized what had happened, the Maltese regiment promptly threw down their arms, refused to fight and were taken prisoner. Other Franco-Neapolitan guns were stationed along the beach and provided with furnaces ready to fire red hot shot at the British squadron which had been sighted beating back from Ponza. However, adverse weather conditions put paid to the squadron's return.

It was now only a matter of time. Lowe capitulated a few days later and surrendered the island, the forts, the artillery, the ammunition and all the stores to the French. He and his troops were shipped off to Sicily. Saliceti could not believe what had happened, landing on Capri was achievement enough, let alone its capture. When it came to matters military, Lowe just wasn't in the same league as Murat.

The following year Saliceti died in uncertain circumstances –

as common with men who plied his trade, it was said to be poisoning. When Napoleon learnt of this he remarked, "His name was worth an army of a hundred thousand men to me."

Colonel Hudson Lowe arrived in Sicily during the planning of an expedition against Naples. When asked for his advice he recommended that Suzzarelli should be consulted! Yet in spite of everything, Lowe continued for the next two or three years to indulge in a bit of well-intentioned espionage and to lead his Corsican Rangers on expeditions to capture various of the Ionian Islands.

In 1812 he was promoted full colonel and sent to Russia and Sweden where he helped in the raising of another troop of apparent misfits, this time of prisoners and deserters from the German Confederation. You well may ask what he thought he was doing but, in retrospect, his activities were steadily making him the inevitable candidate for the governorship of St Helena when the time came. He was spreading himself around, making contacts in the highest places he could worm his way into and continuing with his intelligence work. Somehow or other all this got him attached to Blücher's staff. He was at Blücher's side during the final battles through France of 1813-14. Thus, as the only British officer attached to the Prussians, he was sent to London with the news of Napoleon's defeat and first abdication. He could scarcely believe his good fortune: he was created a Knight Commander of the Bath, and the contacts he had built up with the allied armies won him the Prussian Order of Merit, the Russian Order of St George and mention in the honours lists of several other countries. Not unexpectedly he kept all his contacts on the boil with regular correspondence.

Napoleon, however, didn't agree with Lowe's worth as an aide to Blücher. Speaking to O'Meara, he said:

> "It appears that the Governor was with Blücher, and was the writer of some official letters to your Government, describing the

operations of 1814. I drew his attention to them the last time I saw him, and asked if he was their author. He said he was. I told him they were full of falsehoods and nonsense. He shrugged his shoulders, appeared confused and replied that he believed them true. If those letters were the only accounts he sent, he betrayed his country."

In the summer of 1814 Sir Hudson was quartermaster-general to the British army in The Netherlands with the rank of major-general. It was an important appointment as he was responsible for all aspects of provisioning the army – food, accommodation, armaments, everything an army would need when going to war. When Wellington arrived in April 1815 to take command, he and Lowe did not see eye-to-eye and Major-General Sir Hudson Lowe, KCB, was off, via Genoa, to the south of France where we first made his acquaintance.

After Napoleon's death, the Duke of Wellington offered his opinion of Sir Hudson Lowe, Governor of St Helena: "he was a very bad choice; he was a man wanting in education and judgment. He was a stupid man; he knew nothing at all of the world, and like all men who knew nothing of the world, he was suspicious and jealous."

* * *

And now, *mon ami(e)*, I hope I have been able to cast a glimmer of light on the character of the man who was chosen to be General Bonaparte's keeper during the last five years of his life. Opinions on his worth are polarized, but whichever pole you choose to sit on, Sir Hudson Lowe certainly had a profound influence on Napoleon's well-being and health.

~8~
Regulations, vexations and spiteful tricks

(APRIL – MAY, 1816)

HMS *Phaeton* had arrived on Easter Sunday obliging Lowe to remain on board for another twenty-four hours before proceeding to the Castle where, with all the customary ceremony, he was installed as governor. A message was then sent to Longwood informing them that the new governor would visit General Bonaparte at nine o'clock the next morning.

With Sir Hudson safely installed, the time has come to have a look at the governance of the island as this was to play a significant part in Napoleon's later political management.

The Honourable East India Company had been in unbroken possession of St Helena, under Royal Charter, since 1673. When the Government decided to send Napoleon to the island in 1815 they came to an arrangement with the Company whereby the governor was to be nominated by the Crown but appointed by the Company, and the Company would bear an annual expense equivalent to the average of the preceding three years. Any expense over and above this arising from keeping Napoleon in safe custody was to be borne by the Government.

Before Lowe's arrival the governance of the island was a relatively straightforward matter: Colonel Wilks was the governor appointed by the East India Company, Admiral Sir George Cockburn was in command of the St Helena Naval Station with responsibility for Napoleon, and General Sir George Bingham was in command of the British troops (but not the St Helena Foot

Regiment or the St Helena Artillery). When Lowe appeared on the scene he did so as both civil governor, responsible for the civil government of the island, and military governor, answerable to the British Government for the safe custody of General Bonaparte. What he most certainly did not have was any authority over the St Helena Naval Station, and this included the naval surgeons, be they on board a ship or on dry land. Sir George Cockburn was the admiral in command and all the naval surgeons were answerable to him or his successors. Much though this annoyed Lowe there was absolutely nothing he could do about it – or was there?

Lowe's first visit to Longwood was a complete disaster. Attended by Sir George and a ridiculous number of staff he arrived somewhat before the allotted hour, ignorant of the fact that Napoleon had never in his imperial life received anyone at such an inconvenient hour. (Lowe didn't ask, did he? Or send someone to enquire if it would be convenient? No, *he* was the governor! – and Sir George kept quiet.) Then, as if to make sure that the new governor was aware of local conditions, Longwood chose that moment to launch a display of the weather it could summon up when it put its mind to it. The rain came sheeting down to the accompaniment of a storm force wind which ensured that not one of the huddled group stood the remotest chance of staying dry. The Governor was informed that Napoleon was indisposed and was not receiving visitors that morning. The misery enveloping the party deepened and Lowe, suppressing his anger, squelched up and down in front of the drawing room windows collecting enough clay on his shoes to bring him to a halt. At length he demanded of the door-keeper when on the next day might he be introduced. Two o'clock was the time ordained.

At the appointed hour the next afternoon the same, considerably drier, party again arrived at Longwood. While waiting in the dining room, Sir George said that he would introduce the Governor, this being, he thought, the correct manner for handing over responsibility for the prisoner. For this reason, they would enter the drawing room together. Lowe agreed. After a minute or two, the door opened and the Governor was called for. At the word 'governor' Lowe jumped to his feet, was into the doorway and announced by the valet, Noverraz, before the Admiral had time to collect himself. The door was then closed and Sir George was refused entry as his name had not been called.

Napoleon and Lowe talked, mostly in Italian, for about a quarter-of-an-hour after which the officers of the governor's staff were introduced.

I am not quite sure how this fiasco with Sir George came about. It could have been orchestrated by Napoleon himself because he was inwardly seething at the restrictions imposed upon him by Sir George, or perhaps because he wanted to see Lowe alone believing he would be able to get on well with him. Napoleon himself blamed Sir George, as he explained to O'Meara a day or two later when he brought him some newspapers. (Newspapers arrived from all over the world in incoming ships and were eagerly consumed by the islanders, none more so than Napoleon.)

Napoleon asked how he had come by them.

"The Admiral lent them to me."

"I believe he feels he was rather ill-treated when he came here with the new governor. What does he have to say about it?"

"He considers he was insulted. He was certainly greatly offended."

"But he didn't let Bertrand know that he wished to see me."

"No," O'Meara replied, "because he wanted to introduce the new governor in an official manner, and believed that as he was to act in that capacity he didn't have to be announced."

"Nevertheless, he should have sent word by Bertrand that this is what he had in mind. But," Napoleon continued, "he wished to get me off on the wrong foot with the new governor, which is why he persuaded him to come here at nine o'clock in the morning, well-knowing that I never had, nor ever would, receive anybody at that hour. It is a pity that a man who is really talented – for I believe him to be a very good officer in his own service – should have behaved towards me as he has done."

O'Meara valiantly stood up for his superior officer, saying he was perfectly convinced Sir George had never had the slightest intention of insulting him or of embroiling him with the Governor. Napoleon, though, continued to accuse him of a variety of slights and lack of respect – ignoring the little kindnesses, such as sending him newspapers on their arrival at the risk of incurring Lowe's displeasure. The trouble was that the complete injustice of his status as a prisoner-of-war was eating into Napoleon's very soul and he was unable to look with equanimity on any shape or form of British authority. He might be General Bonaparte to the Governor and all his hangers-on, but to the loyal French banged up in Longwood he was the Emperor Napoleon and was treated as such.

In the weeks that O'Meara had so far been Napoleon's doctor the professional relationship had developed into as genuine a friendship as could be. He enjoyed the Emperor's confidence in the way that only a doctor can and, just as important if not more so in the present situation, he had earned Napoleon's trust. He enjoyed a position unique among the British officers. Regrettably, this relationship with Napoleon and, indeed, his status at Longwood was to be the source of much malignant misunderstanding.

Lowe lost no time in imposing his authority and in the last week of April many new regulations began to appear: Major Gorrequer and other officials went round the shopkeepers in Jamestown ordering them to deny credit to the French and to sell them things only for ready cash; if they disobeyed they would be fined the amount of the loan or whatever other punishment the Governor thought fit to impose. Added to that, the shopkeepers were forbidden to have any form of communication with the French without special permission from the Governor or risk being thrown off the island. This mightily upset Napoleon when he came to hear about it.

And it was not only the civilians who were affected. The officers of the 53rd, in the habit of calling on Fanny Bertrand, who was Irish, started getting hints that these visits were displeasing to the new authorities. Indeed, so heavy were the hints that they decided to go to Hutt's Gate and, *en masse*, take their leave of Madame Bertrand as, in their own words, it was impossible for men of honour to comply with the new regulations. Sentries were posted in all directions and were ordered to report the names of all callers. On one occasion, O'Meara's orderly was delivering medicines for Bertrand's servant who was desperately ill. O'Meara had attached a label with instructions for taking the medicine written in French, but as the sentry couldn't read French he tore it off before allowing the bottle to enter. Longwood didn't escape either, having to endure several more sentries scattered around the house and grounds.

Lowe, who really didn't know where to set the limits, in person closely questioned everyone who had already talked to General Bonaparte or to members of his suite. And to cap it all, everyone who visited Hutt's Gate or Longwood in the future had to make a report either to the Governor or to Sir Thomas Reade of the conversations they had had with the French. The reasonably sociable and friendly atmosphere of the island was no more. It was a situation that went from bad to worse when Lowe began to play at espionage again, this time more successfully than on Capri – not that he had learnt a lesson, just that he was dealing with a different sort of people who, if they didn't toe Sir Hudson's line, would lose their jobs, their chances of promotion, their very freedom.

But besides those regulations that affected everybody, both London and the Governor were busy finding ways to unsettle the General's life. Among the first to appear was a directive from Lord Bathurst for Napoleon's domestics to sign: Did they wish to stay on the island serving their master? If so, they would agree to submit to the same restrictions as were imposed on Bonaparte and his suite. The directive had been badly translated and some of the domestics contacted Sir Thomas Reade for clarification. His answers made it appear that if they signed they would be compelling themselves to stay on the island during Bonaparte's lifetime. Despite the threat, they all signed. This directive was really nothing but a blatant attempt to get rid of loyal servants so that Lowe could introduce his own people to spy on the goings-on at Longwood.

Lowe, on his own initiative, next resorted to a thoroughly spiteful act by interfering with the selection of newspapers sent up to Longwood. Previously, a regular run of some papers as well as odd numbers of others had been sent, but Lowe chose to send only a few odd issues of the Bourbon-leaning *Times* and an occasional issue of the *Courier*. This was not just spiteful, it amounted to mental cruelty and caused considerable distress to those with relatives in France. Indeed, as O'Meara said of the arrival of both letters and newspapers: "A line of writing from Europe is, at Longwood, a treasure above all price." It also disturbed Napoleon as it announced the passing of one era at Longwood and the arrival of another in which humanity was to be cast aside.

Not only was Lowe hell bent on inconveniencing and irritating his prisoner, he was also intent on humiliating him. So, when Lady Moira, wife of the Governor-General of India, was staying at Plantation House he sent an invitation to General Buonaparte (the British Government chose to insult Napoleon by spelling his name in this way), via his Grand Marshal, to come to the House to meet her. Napoleon simply told Bertrand not to answer it. To send such an invitation, knowing that, if he accepted, he would have to go under guard, was a gross insult.

However, the Governor was not done yet. He, like Admiral Cockburn, demanded the twice-daily visual proof of Napoleon's physical presence on the island. But at the start of May, with the approach of winter, the weather became extremely wet and foggy with a high wind, keeping Napoleon indoors. He was feeling low and out of sorts with "a mental condition in consequence of the treatment I receive." Captain Thomas Poppleton, the orderly officer, did not get so much as a glimpse of him for several days.

Even though he had the assurance of the other residents of Longwood that they had heard Napoleon's voice, Lowe wouldn't trust them. He wrote to Bertrand insisting that the orderly officer must see the General every day. He, himself, regularly came up to the house, wandered around, looked in windows and, not one to waste time, laid down the plan of a new ditch to "stop the cattle trespassing" – so he said!

Eventually his persistence paid off and he was admitted to the bedroom for a quarter-hour interview with Napoleon who was in a state of *déshabillé*. During the course of this, the Governor proposed that Napoleon should dismiss O'Meara and take his (Lowe's) physician instead. He got a very frosty answer, but so desperate was he that he repeated the proposal and even turned at the door to try again – he just had to know the true state of Napoleon's health. Were O'Meara's bulletins truthful or overstating the case? Were the reports he received from members of staff or from visitors reliable, based on rumour or simply fabrications? His dispatches to London had to make it clear that General Bonaparte was in the best of health or, if he was not very well, that it was nothing that could be attributed to the climate of St Helena. How was he to manipulate the truth if he didn't know what that was?

The physician Lowe was referring to was Alexander Baxter who, besides his job as Deputy Inspector of Hospitals, was head of the Governor's medical staff, but not attached to him as his personal physician. O'Meara had met him and reckoned, as he told Napoleon, that he seemed a decent sort and was generally regarded as a talented man of science. Although Napoleon would have nothing to do with him as a stooge of the Governor, when Baxter came to Longwood as a private individual, he was pleased to receive him and greeted him with a smile, "Well, *signor medico*, how many patients have you killed in your time?" Baxter took this in the spirit intended and they got on quite amicably for nearly an hour.

The day after his visit to Napoleon, the Governor decided to have a go at his Grand Marshal. He addressed him in a voice of contemptuous authority, beginning with an attack on the French residents whom he accused of making a great many unjustified complaints. Taking everything into consideration, he said, they were well treated and should be thankful for it. Instead, they abused the little kindnesses they were shown and took advantage of the situation whenever they could. Bertrand, understandably, took an extremely dim view of it all.

Without a doubt, the Governor had got under Napoleon's skin. At nine o'clock the next morning Marchand was sent to fetch O'Meara and, taking him through the back way, showed him into the bedroom where Napoleon was lying on an old-fashioned sofa covered with a white longcloth, looking sad and troubled. He was dressed in his white morning gown, white all-in-one trousers and stockings; his shirt collar was open. On his head was a chequered red headscarf. At the foot of the sofa was a small round table with some books on it, others lay strewn around.

Above the mantelpiece hung a portrait of Marie Louise and four or five of the young Napoleon; a little to the right hung a miniature of the Empress Josephine. At the foot of the sofa facing him was another portrait of Marie Louise, as empress, with her son in her arms. A few other treasures, including the alarm chamber-watch of Frederick the Great, were scattered around the room. His little camp bed with its green silk curtains – memories of Marengo and Austerlitz – stood in a corner on a carpet which had once graced the floor of a lieutenant of the St Helena artillery. All the furnishings were dejected and sad with nothing left of former imperial glory except a magnificent washstand with a silver basin and water-jug.

After a few unimportant questions asked in both French and Italian, Napoleon began – and the conversation that follows is vitally important to the future assessment of O'Meara's conduct and the search for the answer to our first question:

"You know that it was in consequence of my application that you were appointed to attend upon me. Now I want to know from you precisely and truly, as a man of honour, what situation do you see yourself as being in; do you see yourself as my surgeon, as M. Maingaud was, or do you see yourself as the surgeon of a prison-ship and its prisoners? Do you have orders to report to the Governor every trifling occurrence or illness or what I say to you? Give me a truthful answer. How do you see yourself?"

"I see myself as your surgeon, and to attend on your suite. I have received no orders other than to make an immediate report should you be taken seriously ill, so that I may seek advice and help from other physicians without delay."

"Having first obtained my consent to call upon these others," Napoleon was quick to jump in, "is that not so?"

O'Meara said it was so.

Napoleon then went on: "If I was in a prison where I knew the governor to be a spymaster and you were its surgeon with orders to report my conversations to him, I would never consult you again – but don't think for one moment that I do take you for a spy," he hastened to add as soon as O'Meara began to protest. "On the contrary, I have never had the least occasion to find fault with you. I have a friendship for you and hold your character in high esteem; indeed, I couldn't have given you greater proof of this than I have done by asking you candidly for your own assessment of your situation. Being an Englishman, you might just have given me the answers I was wanting."

The Irishman made no comment. A moment or two later, Napoleon returned to his theme.

"During those few days when I was melancholic and

distraught, the Governor wanted to send me his physician. His messages came under the pretext of enquiring after my health. But it's the bad weather and the way they treat me. I told Bertrand to tell him I hadn't sufficient confidence in his physician to take anything from his hands, and if I really were ill I would send for you. And to let him know that anyway a physician was useless in such cases; I only wanted to be left alone."

At this point Napoleon became extremely emotional. "I understand he proposed sending an officer into my bedroom to see me if I didn't come out. Any person," O'Meara had never seen Napoleon quite so angry, "who tries to force his way into my apartment shall be a corpse the moment he enters. If he ever eats bread or meat again, I am not Napoleon. This I am determined about; I know I shall be killed afterwards – what else can be done? I have faced death too many times to fear it.

"The Governor might then write home to his Government that '*Buonaparte*' was killed in a brawl. I told him this and to leave me alone and not torment me with his hateful presence. I have seen Prussians, Tartars, Cossacks, Calmucks, but never before have I seen so ill-favoured and forbidding a countenance. He bears the devil's imprint on his face.

"I have had no reason to complain of the Admiral," Napoleon continued, "he may have treated me roughly, but he never behaved in such a manner as this '*Prussian*'. The Admiral has never asked a second time to see me when told I was unwell or undressed. As he well knows, I might not go out, but I am still to be found."

[Napoleon was so convinced that Lowe would attempt to force an entry into his room that, for a short time after Admiral Cockburn left the island, he kept four or five pairs of loaded pistols and some swords at the ready.]

The next day Napoleon returned to the subject of how O'Meara saw his situation on the island.

"According to the strict letter of our conversation yesterday,"

O'Meara responded, "it would be impossible for me to answer any question addressed to me about you or your affairs, whether by the Governor or anyone else.

"Furthermore, since I arrived, I have been used as middle man for communication between yourself and the authorities on the island which I hope I have carried out to your satisfaction."

"Are you to be my surgeon," Napoleon replied, "or 'surgeon to the galley slaves'. Are you expected to report what you see and hear?"

"I am your surgeon in whom I hope you may place your confidence. I am not a spy, I am not a 'surgeon to the galley slaves'. I feel obliged to report only matters that conflict with my loyalty as a British officer.

"But total silence in this regard is impossible if you wish me to maintain any kind of workable communication with the Governor or any other English persons on the island."

"All I ask of you is that you act like an honourable man, as you would do were you surgeon to Lord St Vincent [who, as Admiral Sir John Jervis won the naval battle of Cape St Vincent in 1797]. I do not want to bind you to silence, or to prevent you repeating any gossip you may hear from me. But I do want to stop you being cajoled by this Governor into unintentionally becoming a spy. Your duty, after that to your God, is owed to your own country and sovereign, and after that to your patients."

This second conversation on the subject brings home even more decisively than the first just where O'Meara saw his responsibilities and loyalties to lie as Napoleon's surgeon.

The next flurry of regulations was announced in a proclamation prohibiting "any person from receiving or being the bearer of any letters or communications from General Buonaparte, the officers of his suite, his followers or servants, of any description, or to deliver any to them, under pain of being arrested immediately and dealt with accordingly."

Lowe had, it seemed, a bottomless reservoir of ideas for rubbing the French up the wrong way. Napoleon unburdened himself to O'Meara yet again:

"This Governor," he said, "*è un imbecile.* He asked Bertrand the other day, if he (Bertrand) had ever asked any of the passengers bound for England whether they intended to visit France because, had he done so, he must not do so again. Bertrand said that he certainly had and had, moreover, asked one or two of them to tell his relatives that he and his family were in good health. But, says this imbecile, you must not do so again.

"'Why?' asks Bertrand. 'Hasn't your government allowed me to write as many letters as I like – and can any government deny me the freedom of speech?'

"Bertrand," Napoleon continued, "should have answered that even galley slaves and prisoners under sentence of death were allowed to enquire after their relatives."

Napoleon was lost in thought for a moment, then, "Have you any galley slaves in England," he asked.

"No," said O'Meara, interpreting his words literally, "but we do have some condemned convicts working at Portsmouth and elsewhere."

"Then he ought to have been made their keeper. It would be exactly the sort of office that would suit him."

Having feelingly referred to Lowe as an imbecile, Napoleon further illustrated the point by detailing the stupidity of the security arrangements on the island, such as requiring him to be accompanied by an officer whenever he wanted to venture outside the Longwood boundaries.

"It's all right to keep me away from the town and the coast; I wouldn't want to go there anyway. All that is needed for my security is for the coastline to be well guarded. Let him place his pickets round the island close to the shore – which would be easy for him to do with the number of men he has – and in communication with each other and it would be impossible for me to escape. Couldn't he also put a few horsemen on patrol when he knows I'm going to ride out? He could put them on the hills or where he likes, without letting me know anything about it. I would never show that I'd seen them.

"Can't he do this without obliging me to tell Poppleton that I want to ride out – not that I have anything against Poppleton; I love a good soldier of any nation. [Poppleton was the only orderly officer to have the honour of dining with Napoleon.] It's simply that I will not do anything which may lead people to think I am a prisoner – I have been forced here contrary to the law of nations, and I will never recognize their right in detaining me. My asking an officer to accompany me would be a tacit acknowledgement of it. My health dictates that I ride seven or eight leagues daily, but I will not do so with an officer or a guard over me."

And, as Lowe was worried he might manage to get on board a ship, Napoleon continued: "Can't they simply impose additional restrictions when ships arrive; and above all not allow ships to sail until my actual presence is confirmed, without inflicting such useless, and because useless, vexatious restrictions?"

At the end of the month a ship arrived from England with some French newspapers on board which Sir George handed to O'Meara before reading them himself.

"Who gave you those papers?" Napoleon asked.

"The Admiral. He told me to give them to Bertrand, but he really meant them for you." Much less welcome was the news, which the Governor sadistically told O'Meara to be sure to pass on to General Buonaparte, that a Bill (Bonaparte's Detention Bill) had been brought before Parliament to give legality to his detention on St Helena and to provide the necessary funds for his upkeep.

"Did it meet with any opposition?" asked Napoleon.

"Scarcely any." This amounted to no more than protests entered by Lord Holland and His Royal Highness Prince Augustus

Frederick, the Duke of Sussex.

Was Napoleon to be deprived even of hope?

* * *

And now, *mon ami(e)*, you will see that the Duke of Wellington was correct in his opinion that Sir Hudson Lowe was a very bad choice of governor. You will remember that one of the reasons the British Government chose him was because his lowly beginnings in life would render him less susceptible to Napoleon's charms. And they were correct about that all right! Wellington was again on the ball when he said that Sir Hudson was a jealous man, and is it not written in the *Song of Solomon* (**8**, 6), "jealousy is as cruel as the grave"? Lowe was damned well going to show this upstart emperor who was boss. All his spiteful little tricks had an adverse effect on Napoleon's peace of mind and, ultimately, on his physical health. And O'Meara made it plain just where his duties and his loyalties lay – he was an honourable man.

~9~
A view round the bend

(JUNE – AUGUST, 1816)

On the morning of June 17, 1816, O'Meara sighted the frigate, HMS *Newcastle*, 60 guns, beating up to windward and, fetching his glass, brought her to Napoleon's attention. Well he might, as she was bearing three passengers of potential significance to Napoleon's existence on St Helena. The most important was Rear-Admiral Sir Pulteney Malcolm, Sir George's replacement in command of the St Helena Naval Station. The other two were the Commissioners appointed by the Russian and French Governments to look after their country's interests with regard to Napoleon. A third commissioner, representing Austria, arrived the next day on board the *Orontes*, 36 guns. Prussia, the fourth of the Allied powers, chose not to be represented.

The Commissioners were a mixed bag. Their main purpose was to assure themselves of Napoleon's continued presence on the island, which they contrived to do, quite successfully, without ever setting eyes on the person of General Bonaparte. Their other function was to keep an eye on his English guardians and report to their masters on their behaviour.

The French Commissioner, well known to Napoleon, could have been a character from a Gilray cartoon. He was the Marquis of Montchenu, a member of the *ancien régime* with a considerable military background who had become an *émigré* in 1792. He was devoted to the French royal family and had made no secret of the fact that his greatest wish was to be appointed Napoleon's jailer.

Talleyrand brought this wish to fulfilment, knowing full well that no other person would quite so annoy Napoleon. Since he had no diplomatic skills and no languages other than French, Montchenu was at a decided disadvantage in gathering information for his reports which consequently were of little value. He brought with him his secretary, Captain Jean Claude de Gors (he only acquired the nobiliary particle when he became the marquis's secretary – can't let the side down!).

Having made his presence officially known to the Governor at the Castle and wondering what to do next, Montchenu approached a group of officers on the castle terrace.

"If any of you speak French," he addressed himself, quite fortuitously, to O'Meara who was standing among them, "for the love of God make it known to me, for I do not speak a word of English. I have arrived here to finish my days amongst those rocks (pointing to Ladder Hill) and I can't speak a word of the language."

Napoleon was considerably amused when O'Meara told him of the conversation. "The man's a garrulous idiot," he said. "When you've seen Montchenu, you have seen the old nobility of France before the Revolution.

"What stupidity it is," he continued, "to send these Commissioners out here; they will have nothing to do but walk about the streets and clamber up the rocks. The Prussian Government at least has shown more sense and saved its money." Which was the most charitable thing he had had to say about the Prussians for many a long year.

The other two Commissioners both had diplomatic experience but in the case of the Austrian, Baron Stürmer, this only made him think he was more important than he really was. With him came his wife and a botanist, Philippe Welle, neither of whom helped endear him to Lowe. The wife was French and a great admirer of the Emperor, while the botanist brought with him a lock of the King of Rome's hair sent by Marchand's mother who was the King's nurse. Lowe naturally suspected a conspiracy. Breakfasting one morning with O'Meara, Napoleon asked whether Madame Stürmer had ever seen him in Paris. Yes, said O'Meara, she had and would very much like to see him again.

"And what prevents her?" he asked.

"She doesn't think you would receive her, any more than you would receive her husband or the other Commissioners."

"Who told them that? Of course I'm willing to receive them whenever they choose to ask through Bertrand. But all the powers in Europe would not induce me to see them in their official capacity. I shall only receive them as private persons. You know I never refuse to see anybody when asked in the proper way, and especially I should always be glad to see a lady." Still the emperor!

The Russian, Count Balmain, a descendant of a Scottish family, the Ramsays of Balmain who had left Scotland in 1685, was the only one of the three suited by temperament, education and experience to fulfil the role of commissioner, and the only one who took the job to heart. Having been personally appointed by the Tsar, it was as much as his career was worth to make sure his reports were readable and of value, particularly as he knew they would be read carefully by his master and eagerly devoured by his court. Balmain had charm and was possessed of a much-needed sense of humour.

Regrettably, Napoleon's insistence on protocol never did get through to the Commissioners as the Governor always answered their requests with the statement that Bonaparte refused to see any person whatsoever. (Even Balmain's request to see him as a private individual met with this treatment.) At Plantation House one day when the Commissioners had been on the island for four months and were dining there, Balmain remarked that they would be objects of ridicule in Europe once it was known they had never even seen the individual whose presence was the prime object of their mission. Had he been aware of how he was to be treated, Balmain said he would never have left Russia.

Lowe was, however, seriously concerned about the Commissioners since he was afraid that if they had access to Napoleon, their reports might differ from his often dodgy ones and show him (Lowe) in a bad light. He was also highly suspicious that either Bertrand or Las Cases, or both, were in cahoots with the Commissioners hatching some sort of a plot against him.

Admiral Sir Pulteney Malcolm did not meet Napoleon until the twentieth when he and Captain Henry Meynell, flag captain of the *Newcastle*, were presented by Lowe. Malcolm, a handsome man with engaging manners, made quite an impression on Napoleon. So much so that the next day he enthused to O'Meara:

"Ah, there is a man with a really pleasing face, open, intelligent, frank and sincere. There is the face of an Englishman. I never yet saw a man of whom I so immediately formed a good opinion as of that fine soldier-like veteran. He carries his head erect, and speaks out openly and boldly what he thinks, without being afraid to look you in the eye. His physiognomy would make anyone want to further their acquaintance, and would make even the most suspicious have confidence in him." What on earth had got into the General? Maybe though, this was simply an outpouring of relief at finding himself in sympathy with the new naval commander; let's hope so.

But had Sir Pulteney let Napoleon down after this eulogy (which gushed on ecstatically), the effect on the General's peace of mind could well have been disastrous. Mercifully the Admiral lived up to expectations. He did everything he could to ease the friction between jailer and prisoner and to make life more bearable for Napoleon. In so doing he inevitably aroused the Governor's suspicions that some sort of conspiracy was being hatched. Evidently his physiognomy was no match for the Governor's suspicious mind.

The *Newcastle* had brought with her several packing cases full of the fourteen or fifteen hundred books Bertrand had ordered at

Funchal on the way out. Their delivery to Longwood sent Napoleon into the seventh heaven, and he immediately set about the cases with hammer and chisel. All night he read and in the morning was found by O'Meara in great good humour, grinning like a Cheshire cat with books scattered all over the floor.

"Ah," he said, pointing to a pile, "what pleasure they have given me. And what a difference. I can read forty pages of French in the time it would take me to understand two in English."

The last days of June were celebrated with yet another clampdown on anyone entering into correspondence or any other form of communication with Napoleon or any of his staff without the authorization of Lowe himself. To do so would be an infraction of the acts of parliament for his safe custody and would bring the full force of the law crashing down on their head. This included furnishing him with money or any other means whatever by which his escape might be furthered. And just to make sure that the General didn't step out of line, Lowe wrote to Bertrand informing him that all communications, written and verbal, with the islanders were prohibited unless he, the Governor, had previously given clearance through the orderly officer.

* * *

July, 1816, opened with a spell of foul weather which prevented Napoleon venturing out. Confined indoors, he occupied himself for several hours each day reading the new books and gathering forgotten dates and other information for the history of his life. Even so, he welcomed any diversion, however brief, and a two-hour visit by the Malcolms did him a power of good. Lady Malcolm, in fact, turned out to be one of only three ladies – the other two were Mrs Skelton and Mrs Balcombe – who came to be on really intimate social terms with Napoleon, visiting him and taking the occasional carriage ride together.

The climate and its effect on life generally couldn't be this bad all over the island, could it? The other side, sheltered as it was from this infernal, eternal cutting wind was where an emperor, if he had to live here in the first place, should find his home. So he told O'Meara to start negotiations with the Governor. And much good did they achieve! When Napoleon suggested other more favourable properties Lowe always had a reason why they were unsuitable. What about a completely new building? Where would the General prefer it? At The Briars. No, too near the town, but what about a new building at Longwood? That cut no ice because Napoleon was hankering after some place where he could enjoy shade, greenery and water (running as opposed to waterlogged). "Let him put me on the Plantation House side of the island, if he really wishes to do anything for me. What is the use of his coming up here proposing things, and doing nothing. His proposals are all a delusion anyway. There is Bertrand's house [the new villa being built at Longwood] not the least advanced since the Governor's arrival."

If not a new building, then how about doing something to the existing Longwood? So, despite Napoleon's expressed unhappiness with the place, Lowe discussed at length with Montholon the acceptability of altering, enlarging and generally improving the place. You will not be surprised to learn that the high points of the improvements came when a billiard table was delivered and when Admiral Malcolm sent up a lieutenant with a party of sailors to erect a tent, made from a sail, to provide some shade. Napoleon did, however, almost win the day when the drawing room caught fire at five o'clock one morning – and no, he was not responsible! It was extinguished in about half-an-hour by Captain Poppleton and members of staff, but if they hadn't stopped it just before it reached the floor above, Longwood would have been a mini Moscow.

Napoleon, though, still had high hopes elsewhere:

"I am of the opinion that as soon as the affairs of France are settled, the English Government will allow me to return to Europe and end my days in England. I do not believe they are foolish enough to go to the expense of eight millions annually to keep me here when I am no longer to be feared. I am, therefore not very worried about the house." Wasn't it Aeschylus who said "men in exile feed on dreams of hope"?

Nevertheless, if he could get the Governor (with a nudge from Malcolm, perhaps) to move him to a better part of the island, he wouldn't say no, however short a time was left.

In the middle of this housing debate, Lowe revealed his failure to comprehend the mores of the society in which he found himself. Intended as a civility (Napoleon's choice of word; he was feeling unnaturally benevolent towards them that day) the British Government had sent out a shipment of clothing and other articles it considered the exiles might need. Lowe, however, took it upon himself to select those items that should be sent to Longwood.

"Now, if this Governor was possessed of the feelings of a gentleman," Napoleon made *his* feelings known, "he would have sent a list to Bertrand, stating that the English Government had sent a supply of certain articles which it thought we might want, and that if we stood in need of any, we might order such as we pleased. But instead of acting in a manner dictated by the rules of politeness, this jailer converts a civility into an insult, by selecting the items himself and sending them here without consultation and in a contemptuous manner – as if he were sending alms to a lot of beggars or clothing to convicts. His hands soil everything they touch."

And still the impositions continued to proliferate. The ditches Lowe had been planning (to stop the cattle trespassing?) were completed round the garden – they were eight or ten feet deep (which would break the animal's legs should one fall in). And as if this wasn't enough, more pickets had been established and yet more sentries placed, some of whom could be seen by Napoleon if he chose to take a stroll after sunset. "The only thing left undone now is to put sentries on the doors and windows to prevent me going out; but as long as I have a book, I care but little about it." The trouble was that Lowe was haunted by the memory of Capri; he couldn't allow St Helena to suffer a similar fate.

In the middle of the month (July), Lowe descended on Longwood for a long talk with Montholon and O'Meara about the need to cut down the expenses of the establishment which, he complained, were conducted without due regard for economy. He then moved on to Hutt's Gate to show the Grand Marshal a letter from Lord Bathurst which ordered that the expenses must be reduced to eight thousand pounds per annum in toto. However, an estimate prepared by Denzil Ibbetson, Head of the Commissariat Department on the island, came to a little over nineteen thousand pounds per annum. Lowe then wrote to Montholon demanding twelve thousand pounds a year for the maintenance of Napoleon and his suite, saying that he had already been told by both Napoleon and Montholon himself that he (Napoleon) had adequate funds at his disposal in various parts of Europe.

Two days later the argument was renewed when the Governor and Admiral Malcolm, attended by Sir Thomas Reade and Major Gorrequer, neither of whom took part in the discussion, arrived at Longwood seeking an interview. They wanted to discuss details with General Bonaparte himself, not with his staff. Napoleon, attended by Bertrand, Montholon and Las Cases and his son, happened to be taking a stroll around the garden and was far from pleased at being seen since this meant he could no longer use the excuse of being in the bath not to receive them.

The 'interview', which lasted about half-an-hour, took place in the garden and ended most unpleasantly. Both parties showed their considerable agitation and there was much flinging about of arms. Only Sir Pultney, a disinterested participant, remained calm. On being dismissed, the Governor simply turned on his heel and, without saluting the General, walked over to where O'Meara and

Poppleton were standing. They had witnessed, though not overheard, the whole nasty business.

"General Bonaparte has been very abusive to me. I had to leave him rather abruptly, telling him, '*Vous êtes malhonnête, Monsieur*'." So saying, he mounted his horse and galloped away.

The Admiral removed his hat, made his bow and took his leave looking troubled and thoughtful. It was evident that the interview had, indeed, been very unpleasant.

The next day Napoleon explained to O'Meara why the 'interview' had grown so heated. From the start, he said, the Governor had put his back up by having the audacity to say he had changed nothing on the island since his arrival.

"I have come up to justify myself; in fact I have come up two or three times previously but was told you were in the bath."

"No Sir, I was not in a bath, but I ordered one on purpose not to see you. In endeavouring to justify yourself you make matters worse."

"You do not know me, but if you did you would change your mind."

"Know you, Sir," Napoleon answered, " How could I know you? People make themselves known by their actions; by commanding in battles. You have never commanded in battle. You have never commanded any but vagabond Corsican deserters, Piedmontese and Neapolitan brigands. I know the name of every English general who has distinguished himself, but I never heard of you except as a *scrivano* (clerk) to Blücher or as a commandant of brigands. You have never commanded or been accustomed to men of honour."

"I did not ask for this job of governor."

"No, such employments are not sought, they are given by governments to men who have dishonoured themselves."

"I only did my duty, and you ought not to blame me for that; I was only acting according to my orders."

"So does the hangman! Besides, I do not believe that any government could be so mean as to give such orders as you yourself cause to be executed." [Once again he was beset by benevolent feelings towards the British Government.] "If you wish," Napoleon continued, " and choose not to send me anything to eat, I would go over and dine with the brave officers of the 53rd. I am sure there is not one of them who would refuse to give a plate at the table to an old soldier."

Napoleon then brought up the subject that really distressed him: "That iniquitous parliamentary Bill decreed that I was to be treated as a prisoner, but you have treated me worse than a condemned criminal, or as a galley slave." [Napoleon certainly had a thing about galley slaves!] "*They* are allowed to receive newspapers and printed books which you deny me. You may have power over my body, but you have none over my soul.

"You are a *sbirro Siciliano* (Sicilian cop), not an Englishman. Leave, and do not let me see you again until you come with orders to dispatch me, when you will find all the doors thrown open to admit you."

Lowe then admitted he had found his situation so difficult that he had resigned. This inspired Napoleon to respond, "A worse man than yourself could not be sent out, though the appointment is not one that a gentleman would wish to accept."

When he had finished explaining why the 'interview' had been so unpleasant, he continued, "It is not my custom to abuse any person, but that man's effrontery produced bad blood in me, and I had to make my feelings absolutely clear. When he had the impudence to tell me in front of the Admiral that he had changed nothing on the island, I replied, 'Call your aide-de-camp here, and ask him. I will leave it to *him*.' That struck him dumb, he didn't say a thing!"

Napoleon then gave O'Meara permission, should he have the opportunity, to be at liberty to repeat what he had just been told.

Inevitably, rumours of what had been said crept around the island, ably assisted by O'Meara. Inevitably also, O'Meara found himself summoned to Plantation House to throw some light on the matter of Lowe's resignation. The Governor first asked whether General Bonaparte really had told him he had handed in his resignation as governor.

"Yes, he told me you had said so."

"I never said any such thing, nor ever had an idea of it. He has either invented it, or perhaps has mistaken my expressions. I merely said that if the Government did not approve of my conduct, I would resign. I wish you therefore to explain to him that I never said I had resigned, nor that I had any intention of doing so."

The Governor next asked what else General Bonaparte had told him about the 'interview' and, reluctantly, O'Meara gave him an abbreviated and watered down account. Lowe had the answer to that one: although he (Lowe) may not have commanded an army against Napoleon, he had probably done him more mischief than if they had met in the field. The advice and information he had given during and after the Congress at Châtillon (1814) was what had subsequently been acted upon, and was the cause of the General's downfall.

"I should like him to know this; it will give him a reason for his hatred."

Lowe stalked about the room biting his nails, before returning to the matter in hand with some observations on Napoleon's "impolite and indecent language".

"Tell General Bonaparte that he had better watch his behaviour; if he continues with his present conduct, I shall be obliged to take measures to increase the restrictions already in force." (Treated just like a naughty schoolboy. And it was not even as if he was planning to escape through the use of 'indecent language'.)

With the matter of expenses still unresolved, Major Gorrequer came up to Longwood two or three weeks later to continue the discussion with Montholon. They agreed that the Government would pay a monthly sum of one thousand pounds and anything in excess of that must be paid by Napoleon himself either by bills drawn on a banker in Europe or by his friends. The Emperor, said Montholon (who always referred to him by his title), was quite prepared to pay all the expenses so long as he was allowed the means to do so and so long as the necessary correspondence took place in sealed letters. Gorraquer's answer was predictable: no sealed letters would be allowed to leave Longwood.

In consequence, Napoleon was left with no alternative but to dispose of his property and accordingly, with Lowe's agreement, portions of his silver plate were sent at intervals to Jamestown for sale. But first it had to broken up and the imperial arms and eagles cut out and put by to prevent their becoming souvenirs. The money raised was paid directly to Mr Balcombe.

And so life at Longwood and Plantation House continued, with domestic matters requiring much letter writing (if nothing else, it was something to keep their minds occupied) and with Governor and General devising new ways, or reviving old ones, to get under the other's skin. The ploys of most concern, however, were the restrictions and impositions affecting Longwood since they were responsible for Napoleon's refusals to take exercise. He was not a man to be humiliated. O'Meara, with his acceptance by both sides, found himself the carrier of verbal, and sometimes written, remarks and messages though, when he could, he suppressed the more offensive parts of Napoleon's observations. And, inevitably, the happenings at Longwood provided a rich source of rumour for the islanders to feed on.

* * *

And now, *mon ami(e)*, you will appreciate why the circumstances of Napoleon's life on St Helena were wearing him down. They were enough to drive anybody round the bend. Day by day they were taking their toll. If they are allowed to continue they will inevitably harm his physical or mental health, or both. Think of Lowe as a bully, which he undoubtedly was, and that should give you some idea of the damage he was inflicting on Napoleon's health.

~10~
Of lead poisoning and scurvy

(OCTOBER, 1816)

Napoleon always made life difficult for O'Meara when it came to treating whatever was the matter with him. Despite having acquired an almost encyclopaedic knowledge of medical matters by extensive reading and persistent questioning, he maintained he knew his body best and stubbornly refused to take any remedy O'Meara had to offer. When unwell, his practice was to eat nothing, drink plenty of barley water, abstain from wine and ride for twenty miles or so to promote perspiration. "Medicines are fit only for old people!"

Early in October he had the chance to show that he was as good as his word when he was driven by a severe headache to go for a ride for the first time in eight weeks. "But," he grumbled, "the limits are so circumscribed that I cannot ride for more than an hour and for it to do me any good I should ride very hard for three or four."

Shortly afterwards he again woke with a headache, but this time with the addition of a colicky pain in his belly and generally feeling rather unwell. O'Meara wanted him to take a dose of some medicine or other but, true to form, Napoleon said he would cure himself with diet and chicken water. Later in the day, both Gourgaud and Montholon complained of similar symptoms and attributed them to contamination of the wine with lead – a not uncommon happening, usually caused by the deliberate use of litharge (lead monoxide) to reduce the harshness of the wine or unintentionally from contact with lead pipes or containers.

After three days of imperial bellyache, O'Meara tried to persuade Napoleon to take some Epsom salts. He refused and said that if he were not better by the next day he would dose himself with his own medicine. Fortunately, the attacks in all three patients were mild and settled without assistance.

Since the contaminated wine had been among the provisions sent up by Mr Balcombe from the East India Company's stores in Jamestown, a few bottles of claret were borrowed from Captain Poppleton as the 53rd got their wine elsewhere,. However, when the wine committee of the 53rd heard of the disaster, they voted to send a case across to Longwood. This gesture decided Cipriani, now the maître d'hôtel at Longwood, to ask them for a dozen or two more to keep Napoleon's table supplied until the crisis was resolved; he would pay for them either in cash or in kind.

This just showed that, given half a chance, there were people on St Helena who could behave like civilized human beings. But when Lowe heard of these negotiations, he sent for O'Meara who, as always, had been the go-between, and told him he had no business acting in that capacity, thus echoing Gorrequer's opinion that the wine had been sent out for the use of General Bonaparte, and he should bloody well drink the stuff or get nothing else. An explanation of the circumstances, however, satisfied the Governor – he couldn't let it get back to London that he had denied the General access to safe wine; after all there were limits to the hardships he could impose!

Since his arrival on the island, Napoleon had complained of nothing that O'Meara regarded as worth more than a laconic comment, as when he had an attack of 'catarrh' – most likely to have been a contemporary variant of influenza. However, at the end of July he had complained of a slight pain in his right side which in O'Meara's book was nothing to worry about – particularly if it didn't recur. He simply advised Napoleon to have it well rubbed with eau de Cologne and flannel by one of his valets and suggested he took a dose of medicine. Napoleon laughed hollowly at this and patted him on the cheek. It was, though, probably the first niggle of trouble to come.

The problems may at first have been small, but concern over his health began to gather momentum when, at the beginning of October, Napoleon complained bitterly of toothache which had kept him awake for most of the night and left him with a swollen cheek. The cause was a wisdom tooth which was carious, loose and an obvious site of focal infection – a danger to vulnerable tissues elsewhere in the body. Extracting it gave O'Meara little difficulty.

When O'Meara made his routine morning visit a day or two afterwards, Napoleon was still in his bath – nothing unusual about that – however, he was complaining of another of his headaches, only this time with a difference: it was accompanied by a feeling of general uneasiness and a low fever. One look in his mouth told O'Meara, the naval surgeon, all he needed to know. It was the all-too-familiar sight of scurvy, the curse, the death-knell of sailors down the years. There was no mistaking the pale, spongy-looking gums which started bleeding when he touched them; the imperial breath didn't smell too good either!

O'Meara told Napoleon to eat more vegetables and sour milky foods than was his wont, to use acidic gargles and to exercise. There was nothing more he could do for his patient except to complain bitterly to Lowe about the deficiency of vegetables at Longwood. Regrettably, cabbages, peas and, indeed, all vegetables were exorbitantly expensive and not exactly plentiful. The islanders usually sold or bartered their home-grown vegetables to the ships or to the troops stationed on the island. The water-cresses in the Jamestown valley were regarded as suitable only for sailors and the more impecunious of the voyagers arriving in Jamestown. O'Meara had an uphill struggle on his hands.

After two days and still complaining of feeling unwell, Napoleon was convinced that, things being as they were, he couldn't last long – scurvy can take you that way. He assured O'Meara that he had followed all his instructions except for the exercise which, as O'Meara well knew, he was prevented from taking by the restrictions imposed on him. Anyway, you don't recover from scurvy overnight.

With that out of the way, Napoleon changed tack and asked O'Meara to feel his heart. He was worried that he had never felt it beat; could it be defective in some way? O'Meara was likewise stumped but attributed his inability to feel anything to imperial obesity and not to a defective organ. (The stethoscope was still to be invented.) As a sop for Napoleon's anxiety, he told him that quite often when taking his pulse he had found his heart rate to be very slow, rarely exceeding 58 or 60 beats a minute and usually only 54. The Emperor was satisfied.

Incidentally, the stethoscope was invented to overcome the very same problem that O'Meara was having with Napoleon's heart: the fat patient. At the Hôpital Necker in Paris, René Laennec was dissatisfied with his examination of a young lady's heart. Neither percussion nor palpation helped at all on account of her fatness, and her age and sex ruled out putting his ear directly on her chest wall. Instead he rolled a student's notes into a tube and applied one end to the lady's chest and his ear to the other. He was impressed with how much he was able to hear and set about developing this primitive stethoscope into a cylindrical wooden version with suitably shaped ends. (A stethoscope that would be recognized as such today first appeared on the scene in about 1860.) However, Laennec's triumph was not the instrument but what it enabled him to achieve. The second edition of his book (1826) contained detailed descriptions of the diseases of the heart and lungs, systematically working through diagnosis, pathology and treatment. This book has been described as the most important treatise on diseases of the thoracic organs ever written. Alas, Laennec died that same year of tuberculosis of the lungs, the very disease he had done so much to alleviate.

* * *

And now, *mon ami(e)*, you will appreciate that in small ways ill-health was beginning to creep up on Napoleon. The scurvy and the dental problems were the main physical causes so far, but of longer-term significance was the pain in his side. And don't forget the variety of psychological onslaughts on his health. He had been on the island for just one year.

~11~
A rose by any other name…?

(OCTOBER – DECEMBER, 1816)

"One half of all the vexations I have experienced here have arisen over the title by which I am addressed." The regular confrontations over his designation were wearing Napoleon down and he again had a mind to adopt an incognito. Nevertheless, he maintained that his staff were correct to call him the *Empereur Napoléon*, to which, he argued, he was fully entitled:

"I abdicated the throne of France, but not the title of Emperor. Sovereigns generally retain their titles." To address him in writing as General Buonaparte was an insult, and the name 'Napoleon', if he were to be called Napoleon Bonaparte might bring back memories better forgotten. He proposed, therefore, to resolve the situation by adopting another name as, indeed, had been his intention when he abdicated. However, he thought the name he had chosen on that occasion, 'Colonel Meuron', might give offence by denoting military rank, so it would be preferable to take that of 'Baron Duroc', baron being the lowest feudal title. (Marshal Duroc had been Grand Marshal of the Palace and a particularly dear friend of Napoleon's; he was mortally wounded at Bautzen when the front of his abdominal wall was carried away by a ricocheting cannon ball. He lived on for a few hours in sublime agony.)

A simple solution, you might think, to Napoleon's vexation.

O'Meara went immediately to Plantation House with Napoleon's suggestion, written in his own hand but unsigned. Lowe was taken aback: "This is a very important communication. I shall consider carefully whether my terms of reference will allow him to adopt either of the names proposed. I shall forward it to the Government without delay, but he must not use either until I have the sanction of the Government for that purpose. Even so, it would be more satisfactory if it were signed by the person in whose name it is presented. Tell him that I am ready to confer at any time with General Bertrand on the subject."

He then committed these thoughts to paper and told O'Meara to take what he had written back to General Bonaparte. "Do you think he will sign it?" he asked.

"Perhaps he might, particularly if you authorize him to use either of the names."

When O'Meara got back to Longwood, Napoleon explained that it had not been his intention for the Governor to keep the letter. That it was left unsigned was intentional. He simply wanted to make the Governor aware of his views on the subject and to find out whether he would be prepared to meet him half-way. Then, after discussions with Bertrand, he would compose an official letter and sign it.

O'Meara was sent to retrieve the draft document. Lowe returned it, hinting that such a demand pointed to a lack of sincerity on the General's part.

"Tell him," he said, "that by referring this to the British Government, I am not asking permission for General Bonaparte to change his name, but merely seeking to know whether they would recognize such a change."

Napoleon's only response was to ask O'Meara whether the Governor had it in his power to authorize the change. O'Meara didn't know.

"Then, before any further steps are taken, let him reply positively whether he is authorized or not. *Si o no*."

The ship carrying the Governor's despatches on the subject sailed for England in the evening. The only reply His Majesty's ministers ever condescended to make was contained in a scurrilous article in the *Quarterly Review* which Lowe took good care was sent to Longwood as soon as a copy reached the island.

Any charge of lack of sincerity would seem better levelled at the Governor than the Emperor.

* * *

Napoleon's dental health took another downturn when O'Meara found his cheek again to be considerably swollen. Another carious tooth was extracted and O'Meara renewed his antiscorbutic advice, continuing to emphasize the need for exercise as soon as the swelling had subsided to which Napoleon responded with feeling:

"There is either a furious wind with fog which gives me a swollen face when I go out, or when that is wanting, there is a sun which scorches my brains for want of shade. They leave me on purpose here in the worst part of the island." Was he going to reopen the housing debate?

Nevertheless, three days later he did go out in his carriage for the first time in a long while. When he got back, he was obviously pleased with himself and told O'Meara he had followed his prescription and his face was much better.

Unfortunately, the smile was wiped off everyone's faces in the afternoon. At five o'clock, after coming in from a walk, Napoleon sent for O'Meara who found him sitting in front of the fire. He had a headache, was coughing badly and having rigors. His tonsils were swollen, his cheek inflamed and his pulse was racing. He had tonsillitis. O'Meara recommended warm fomentations to his cheeks, a liniment for his throat, warm diluted drinks, a gargle, massage of his feet and total abstinence.

O'Meara looked in again at nine o'clock to find his patient had complied with all of these directions, except the liniment. Not bad going! He now wanted him to take a diaphoretic to make him sweat, but Napoleon preferred to continue with his warm drinks. Either these proved effective or the tonsillitis was running its natural course as he perspired profusely during the night and was much improved the next morning. O'Meara took it upon himself to notify the Governor of this bout of tonsillitis, emphasizing that he attributed it to the violence of the wind and the bleak, exposed situation of Longwood. He was not going to let the opportunity slip by. Lowe surely would want to take some action over a report stating that the captive's illness was brought about by conditions which were in his power to improve.

"The fact is that General Bonaparte wants to get Plantation House," the Governor was not in the mood to play ball, " but the East India Company will not consent to have so fine a plantation given to a set of Frenchmen, to destroy the trees and ruin the gardens." Long live xenophobia!

The improvement of the morning was not, however, to continue. By five o'clock Napoleon had slipped back a bit; the right side of his jaw was considerably swollen, and his tonsils were making swallowing difficult and painful. O'Meara recommended the usual remedies, including a purgative the next morning, but Napoleon would have none of them except his warm drinks and the fomentations.

"I have never taken any medicine since I was a child. I know my own constitution and I know that even a very small dose will produce violent effects. And, moreover, its effects would be contrary to the efforts of nature." O'Meara certainly did have an uphill struggle.

Once again the night brought an improvement and the next morning O'Meara made it plain to his patient that if he persisted with his refusal to take the medicines, he would, in all probability, soon be a dead man should he be attacked by any of the island's endemic diseases. Napoleon's own remedies were totally inadequate for subduing a formidable complaint (not that the available medicines were anything to write home about). But still Napoleon believed it better to do nothing than to take the medicines.

When he was recovered – except for swollen legs, which might have been a hangover from the scurvy – Napoleon had a visit from the Governor enquiring after his health. That topic dealt with, they indulged themselves in their usual squabble over exercise and restrictions, ending with Lowe saying he would consider the General's solution (which he already knew) to the problem of his being so closely guarded when he went out for a ride. He then asked O'Meara to send him a written statement giving his opinion of General Bonaparte's health as he had to prepare a report for the Government.

"In writing it, you must bear in mind that the life of one man is not to be put into competition with the mischief he might cause were he to get loose. And you must recollect that General Bonaparte has already been a curse to the world, and has caused the loss of many thousands of lives. Your position is very peculiar and one of great political importance." O'Meara was being asked to write a politically biased report, and that he would never do.

Throughout the rest of November Lowe took a delight in needling Napoleon in a variety of ways. Thus on the ninth, Napoleon told O'Meara: "That Governor has closed the path to the Company's gardens. Sometimes I used to walk there, as it is the only spot sheltered from the vicious wind, which I suppose he thought was too great an indulgence. But I do not give myself any uneasiness about it, for when a man's time is come he must go. When destiny wills, it must be obeyed."

So O'Meara again wrote to the Governor emphasizing that if Napoleon continued to remain indoors and take no exercise, he would lay himself open to some serious complaint which would, in all probability, prove fatal.

But it wasn't the Emperor who fell foul of the St Helena

climate, it was his *Signor dottore* who developed "a liver complaint, a disease extremely prevalent, and frequently fatal in the island" which makes it reasonable to assume it was hepatitis, although O'Meara himself didn't give it a label.

He had already been feeling unwell for a few days when he asked Dr Maclean, one of the surgeons to the 53rd, to come and bleed him "very profusely". Shortly afterwards he was with Napoleon in his dressing room when he collapsed on the floor. On coming to, he found himself in a chair with a very concerned Napoleon bending over him, loosening his shirt collar with one hand and holding a bottle of vinegar under his nose with the other. He had already removed his cravat and dashed eau de Cologne in his face.

"When I saw you fall," he said, "I thought at first you had slipped, then when you lay still, it seemed it must be an apoplectic fit. But when I saw your face was the colour of death, with your lips white and motionless and no evident respiration, I realized it was either a fit of syncope or that your soul had departed."

At this moment Marchand came in and Napoleon ordered him to bring some orange-flower water, one of his favourite remedies. He then told O'Meara what he had done:

"Did I act correctly?" he asked.

"Yes," replied O'Meara, "you have done everything a surgeon would have done under similar circumstances, except for putting me in a chair; you should have left me lying on the floor."

As O'Meara was leaving the room, he heard Napoleon tell his valet, *sotto voce*, to keep an eye on him in case he had another fit.

* * *

What was arguably one of the cruellest blows Napoleon had to suffer was delivered on the twenty-fifth. Returning to Longwood, O'Meara met the Governor riding up and down the road. When he drew near, Lowe said, with an air of triumph:

"You will meet your friend Las Cases in custody!"

And a few minutes later, sure enough, Las Cases, escorted by the Governor's aide-de-camp, passed by on his way to Hutt's Gate, now part of the military establishment since the Bertrands had moved to their new villa at Longwood. Here he was confined with his son. Las Cases's crime had been to give a letter, written on silk, to one of his servants to take to England – an imbecilic plan if ever there was one as the servant was a slave who could neither read nor write and knew no one in England. Inevitably, the Governor had been told of the plan and, inevitably, the servant was duly examined and sent to prison.

Napoleon, who knew nothing of the letter, was deeply upset at losing Las Cases. "Las Cases," he said, "is the only one of the French who can speak English well, or explain it to my satisfaction. I shall not now be able to read an English newspaper. Madame Bertrand understands English perfectly; but you know one cannot trouble a lady. Las Cases was necessary to me."

Las Cases *et fils* were confined in Hutt's Gate until the end of December and allowed to see no one unless one of the Governor's staff was present. All communication with Longwood was prohibited as Lowe maintained that Las Cases had been the cause of much mischief between Bonaparte and himself. Napoleon was even denied permission to say farewell. "What can he be afraid of? That I would tell him to write to my wife? He will do that anyway. Does he think that Europe is a gunpowder keg, and Las Cases the spark to blow it up?"

However, the Governor just wanted to make his point since he allowed Bertrand and Gourgaud, with Captain Poppleton for company, to visit Las Cases in the Castle on the day of his departure. At breakfast they were left to themselves with only Poppleton, who understood French not at all when spoken by Frenchmen at conversational speed, as supervisor. Afterwards they spent some hours in the large room of the Castle walking up and down one side with Colonel Wynyard and Major Gorrequer on the other. There was every opportunity for letters to be handed over. At about 3pm, father and son embarked on board HMS *Griffon*, sloop-of-war, bound for the Cape of Good Hope. The Governor and members of his staff accompanied them to the quayside.

* * *

And so, *mon ami(e)*, you will appreciate that there was just no let up in the antagonism between Governor and General. It amounted to a relentless day-by-day conflict, and its effects on Napoleon's well-being were beginning to show. And remember that O'Meara had been given no orders other than to make an immediate report to the Governor should Napoleon become seriously ill. Routine reports about the goings-on at Longwood were not on the agenda. And while you're at it, remember also that O'Meara was still an officer in the Royal Navy and as such answerable only to the Commander-in-Chief of the St Helena Naval Station.

~12~
Domestic circumstances

(JANUARY 1 – JULY 4, 1817)

With the dawning of his second New Year in exile General Bonaparte had been on the island for fourteen months. O'Meara wished him a happy New Year. "I hope it will find me better situated. Perhaps I shall be dead, that would be much better," Napoleon then added with a laugh, "worse than this cannot be."

Nevertheless, he was in very good spirits as he distributed the seasonal presents; a handsome snuff-box (from his seemingly inexhaustible supply) for O'Meara, a set of chess-men for Bertrand, unique porcelain pieces for the two countesses, Bertrand and Montholon, and gifts for staff and children.

This display of bonhomie apart, the year got off to an inauspicious start with the first two weeks shrouded in fog so dense that the routine signals from the army camp at Deadwood couldn't be seen, giving rise to interminable squabbles over restrictions, sentries and so on which kept everyone occupied and on their toes and giving Napoleon a severe headache in the process.

However, he did enjoy almost uninterrupted good spirits for the next seven or eight months with few complaints and those mainly of headache and the occasional toothache. By early March, he was taking much more exercise – but only in the form of walking within the confines of Longwood.

Indeed, the wonder is that Napoleon was able to remain as healthy as he did throughout those months considering the conditions endured by anyone living at Longwood – and the staff, too, suffered their fair share of illnesses. At the best of times the drinking water was in short supply since Longwood had no source of its own unlike the estates, such as The Briars and Plantation House, which were favoured with streams running through their grounds. All water for Longwood had to be brought from nearly three miles away and on one occasion during these months Captain Poppleton was compelled to lodge an official complaint that not only was the water becoming scarcer but most of what they did get was sour, turbid and had a decidedly unpleasant taste from being delivered in old wine and rum casks.

When Napoleon left The Briars he had remained on excellent terms with the Balcombes and William saw no harm in supplying Longwood with their provisions on a fairly liberal scale (with no objections from Admiral Cockburn). But this made Sir Hudson suspicious and for once in his life he was right, though he didn't find this out until the Balcombes, considering discretion to be the better part of valour, had left the island. William Balcombe had in fact been working as go-between in the transmission of clandestine correspondence for the French and in negotiating bills for Napoleon. On his return to England he had lived a straightened existence for a few years until he was appointed – by Bathurst of all people! – to the important post of Colonial Treasurer of New South Wales which he filled most ably. (Evidently Bathurst hadn't taken too serious a view of his misdemeanours. Napoleon was his target.)

As time wore on, and despite Balcombe's efforts, shortages and deliveries of food of bad quality were such that Cipriani had to make regular journeys into Jamestown for extra provisions, paying for them with money from the imperial resources. The need grew particularly urgent with the onset of summer when the daily allowance of meat, vegetables and other perishables, carted up to Longwood under the tropical sun, arrived unfit to eat. The Governor refused permission for Cipriani to go down to the valley to buy sheep and vegetables directly from the farmers, although he did allow the Company's farmer to supply Longwood with a couple of calves, at French expense, every month to satisfy Napoleon's partiality for veal.

Although it may seem that Longwood wasn't doing too badly, this was not the case if you were actually living there – and some forty-five people were doing just that. Both Poppleton and O'Meara were regularly complaining to Gorrequer or the Governor about deficiencies, but in truth they all had to lump it. If the food wasn't there, not even the Governor could conjure it up out of thin air.

And provisions weren't the only goods in short supply. Fuel, in the shape of wood and coal (imported from England), was yet another source of complaint, all the more feelingly expressed as June was the middle of the St Helena winter. Montholon pointed out that in Admiral Cockburn's time, they had been given more than double the quantity actually allocated (Balcombe's kindness and Cockburn's blind eye again); if Lowe thought it improper to increase the quantity supplied by the Government, would he kindly authorize the purveyor to increase the amount and the French would pay for it. After some discussion, Lowe gave orders for the allocation to be increased. Napoleon's bath water couldn't be allowed to get cold – even though he might lie in it for two or three hours.

Then there was the state of the Longwood building itself. Alive with rats, the space between the double wooden partitions of the internal walls became a rat's happy playground. At night they invaded the bedrooms. Poisoning them was a bad idea as their bodies couldn't be retrieved and lay where they had fallen – not the most pleasant of smells. To expect the local dogs or cats to do the job was a non-starter as they soon became either indifferent or unwilling hunters when the rats retaliated. So, it was just another inconvenience that, like the rest of the community, they all had to put up with.

The wooden roofs and ceilings were even worse. They were covered with brown paper smeared with a composition of pitch and tar which, in the midday sun melted and ran off to leave gaps for the tropical rains to pour through. Spare a thought for the Countess Montholon who frequently had to get up more than once in the night to move her own and her children's beds to different parts of the room. Any attempt at repair was pointless as the next sunny day and it happened all over again.

Meantime, Admiral Malcolm was doing his best to bring peace and harmony to the Emperor/Governor relationship which lay at rock bottom. He told Napoleon he was mistaken in the Governor, that he was a good man at heart and urged him to let bygones be bygones – had he then been aware of Lowe's comprehensive system of espionage with every smallest detail being reported to him, he might well have been less enthusiastic.

Malcolm did, however, hope that the arrival of Lord Amherst, on his way home from a special mission to China, and of Admiral Sir Robert Plampin, on his way from England to replace Malcolm, might improve matters.

He believed that when the time came it should be the Governor who introduced both new arrivals to Napoleon; indeed, he felt that Lord Amherst was sufficiently distinguished that he should *only* be introduced by the Governor. But when he put this to Napoleon, "I would not receive my own son if he were to be presented by him," was the uncompromising reply. And he wasn't going to budge over the new admiral either. All Malcolm managed to achieve in the end was a souring of the Admiral/Governor relationship as Lowe just couldn't abide the fact that Malcolm enjoyed free access to Napoleon and he didn't. Moreover, Malcolm not only enjoyed the confidence of Napoleon but also had won his affection and friendship.

* * *

The St Helena Turf Club held two race meetings a year (in April and September) on the Deadwood plain which were well-attended high points in the social calendar. Napoleon attended both inaugural meetings in 1817, but at a distance. He walked across to the Bertrands' villa and, from an upper room, had an excellent view of the meeting; he stayed till the end and thoroughly enjoyed himself.

At the meeting itself, also having a good time, were the three Commissioners and Madame Stürmer; they were joined by General Gourgaud. But someone had slipped up as no British officer had been deputed to monitor their conversation. Towards the end of the meeting the group adjourned to the home of Catherine Younghusband, wife of a senior captain in the 53rd, where again they were without surveillance.

The following morning a furious Sir Thomas Reade called on the lady and told her that the Governor should send her off the island for having invited her guests without supervision. She was indeed fortunate to escape punishment as she had been in trouble before when a letter of hers had been found among Las Cases's papers on his arrest. Lowe was also annoyed with the Commissioners who were "mean wretches" for having spoken to Gourgaud when his master (Napoleon) treated them with such contempt by refusing to see them. Reade was indeed a worthy disciple of *his* master.

[The races were inaugurated by Commander the Hon. Henry John Rous, later Admiral and Viscount Dunwich, First Earl of Stradbroke, and a recognized authority on horse racing; he was honorary handicapper of the Jockey Club. Just thought you might be interested.]

* * *

William Pitt Amherst was truly a distinguished visitor. His Uncle Jeffrey, whom he had succeeded to the title of Baron

Amherst, had been commander-in-chief of the army and his father had been adjutant-general and an aide-de-camp to the king. He himself went on to become viceroy of India (an East India Company appointment in those days) and an earl. You may be wondering why I am telling you all this, but who said what and to whom while Lord Amherst was on St Helena troubled Sir Hudson's mind for ages afterwards.

Anyway, the reason for the Amherst Mission had been the injustices and unreasonable demands heaped on the English merchants in Canton by the Chinese mandarins. Lord Amherst was chosen as the British envoy to Beijing to make plain to the Chinese emperor that all this had to stop. Regrettably, the Chinese had not experienced the power of Britain and treated the envoy as an inferior being. Lord Amherst refused to kowtow (bang his forehead nine times on the ground) if admitted to the emperor's presence but said he would bow instead. No compromise could be reached; both sides were mounted on the high horses of empire and proceedings grew steadily more insulting until eventually the Amherst Mission was escorted out of the country and headed off home in their frigate, HMS *Alceste* (originally the *Minerve* captured from the French in1806).

But their troubles weren't over. On the voyage home the *Alceste* struck a rock in the Straits of Gaspar in the Java Sea and sank. There was no loss of life as all personnel were saved by the accompanying Brig, HMS *Lyra* and taken to Batavia where they were transferred to HMS *Caesar*, 80 guns. They arrived at St Helena on June 27 and on the twenty-eighth, accompanied by the Governor, Lord Amherst visited the Bertrands. When Napoleon learned the details of the visit, he was at his most scathing:

"On arriving at the Bertrands with the ambassador," he said, "the Governor merely introduced him as Lord Amherst and then, without sitting down or conversing for a moment like a gentleman, turned about and took his leave, like a jailer or a turnkey who points out his prisoners to visitors, then turns the key and leaves them to get on with it. Having accompanied Lord Amherst, he ought to have remained for a quarter of an hour and then left." Napoleon was punctiliousness itself about observing the correct protocol for the occasion, particularly in court and diplomatic circles.

The next evening when O'Meara found himself among those invited to dine with Lord Amherst at Plantation House, he felt bound to warn him that should he venture up to Longwood with the Governor or any of his staff to see the Emperor, he would most certainly meet with a refusal. This might be construed by some people as an insult but this was the last thing that would be in Napoleon's mind. However, should he visit with only his own staff, O'Meara was in no doubt at all that he would receive a warm welcome. His lordship showed no surprise as he was used to the shenanigans of folk in high places, nevertheless he was grateful for the advice.

On July 1, Lord Amherst, accompanied only by his suite and by Sir Murray Maxwell, FRS, captain of the ill-fated *Alceste*, was received by Napoleon. During the two hours they were alone together Napoleon told him of the effect that Bonaparte's Detention Bill was having on the way he was treated. Amherst showed great concern as, he said, the object of the Bill was not to render worse, but to ameliorate the circumstances of his captivity. He assured Napoleon that he would not fail to make his representations known to the Prince Regent, Lord Liverpool and Lord Bathurst.

Napoleon then had a word with all the members of his lordship's suite; when it came to Captain Maxwell's turn Napoleon reminded him that he (Maxwell) had captured a French frigate off the island of Lissa, in the Adriatic, in 1811, which would make amends for the loss of the *Alceste*! (Either a spot of homework or a tribute to Napoleon's remarkable memory.)

Three days previously HMS *Conqueror*, 74 guns, bearing Rear-

Admiral Sir Robert Plampin to his new appointment as Commander-in-Chief of the Cape and St Helena Naval Stations in succession to Sir Pulteney Malcolm, had sailed into the Jamestown anchorage. On July 3 he, together with his secretary and Captain John Davie of the *Conqueror*, was introduced to Napoleon by Sir Pulteney. That evening O'Meara dined *tête-à-tête* with the Emperor who asked whether he had seen the new admiral and then remarked on the singular difference between the two men:

"Few men," he said, "have so prepossessing an appearance and manner as Malcolm; but the other reminds me of one of those drunken little Dutch *schippers* that I have seen in Holland, sitting at a table with a pipe in his mouth, a cheese, and a bottle of Geneva in front of him."

Sir Pulteney, with his wife, sailed the next day for England aboard the *Newcastle*. The latter, with his 'Lady' Plampin, remained to bring an accession of misery to Longwood.

* * *

And now, *mon ami*(*e*), you understand that the general circumstances of Napoleon's existence on the island were all against him and, each in its own way, contributing to the other baleful influences on his health.

~13~
The Admiral's mistress

(JULY – SEPTEMBER, 1817)

And now, *mon ami(e)*, we are coming to the crunch point of the answer to our first question. Except that Napoleon's health and general fitness were not as good as they had been on his arrival (and you know the whys and wherefores of that), there would appear to be no good reason why life, awful though it may have been for some, should not have proceeded with little fundamental change until Napoleon either died or was removed from the island. However, to truly understand the significance of what I am about to tell you, you must have the key points of the story so far in the front of your mind:

- Napoleon gave himself up to the Royal Navy. He was not captured.
- His personal doctor at the start of his exile, Barry O'Meara, was a serving officer in the Royal Navy and as such reported only to the admiral in command of the St Helena Naval Station. It was the admiral's responsibility to decide what action to take over the reports O'Meara made to him.
- If O'Meara made a special report on Napoleon's health to the Governor, it was only to be with his patient's permission; nevertheless, there had not as yet been any serious medical crisis where such a consideration would come into play (except for the attack of tonsillitis when O'Meara's motives had not been those of the seriousness of the illness).
- Napoleon was no ordinary patient since his well-being, or

otherwise, had political implications which, it might be argued, could compromise 'patient confidentiality'.

- The Governor was responsible for sending back to London reports on the state of affairs on the island with particular reference to Napoleon's activities and state of health. Sir Hudson Lowe was quite obsessed with the idea that these reports, especially those relating to Napoleon's well-being, should be painted in glowing colours to show what an excellent job he, the governor, was doing. Consequently, he considered he had to be aware of, and to censor, if needs be, all information leaving the island.
- The Governor had no authority over O'Meara, although it was something he would give his right arm for.

* * *

We must now step back in time by a few weeks to join Admiral Sir Robert Plampin on board his flagship, the *Conqueror*, in Portsmouth harbour. Early on the morning of departure he had ordered a ship's boat to make for a landing place on the Isle of Wight. It returned, just as the *Conqueror* was getting under way, with a passenger. Nothing peculiar about that – admirals were a law unto themselves. What made it most unusual, not to say highly irregular, if not unique, was something that did not escape the notice of the entire ship's company. The passenger joining the fifty-five-year-old bachelor admiral was a lady and, to the surprise of all on board, she joined the ship as Lady Plampin. Nevertheless, by being smuggled on board in this manner she naturally enough set tongues wagging. After all, no one supposed for a moment that the Admiralty would deny passage to the wife of an admiral!

The *Conqueror*'s surgeon was the extremely experienced John Stokoe who had joined the Royal Navy in 1794 as surgeon's mate and been present at the bombardment of Copenhagen and, on board HMS *Thunderer*, 74 guns, at the battle of Trafalgar. He was offered the post of surgeon on the *Conqueror* while she was still fitting out at Portsmouth and he accepted even though he knew where she was going and how long the tour of duty would be. He had completed twenty-one years of service and would soon be entitled to his retiring pension. He was thus sufficiently senior to have chosen any posting he liked. Was it, perhaps, the chance of seeing and even meeting the ex-emperor that decided him to sail on the *Conqueror*? But, whatever the reason, being so close to receiving his pension, he was unlikely to blot his copybook.

Yet that is precisely what he did at the start of the voyage when he refused to sit at table with the lady – not the best way to get yourself into your commanding officer's good books. Admiral Plampin neither forgave nor forgot the insult. The ship's officers believed that Stokoe's behaviour indicated that he knew more than, in fact, he did; nevertheless, it fuelled the speculation a hundredfold. Did their surgeon know something they didn't? No he didn't, but why let that ruin their sport?

News of the forthcoming arrival of the *Conqueror* had been brought from the Cape a few days earlier by the 14-gun brig-sloop HMS *Podargus*, with the added information that the new admiral was accompanied by a woman – this alone set the ladies' whiskers twitching. The arrival of any vessel aroused their curiosity, but to have their attention drawn to one particular woman – well, that was something quite else!

Consequently, when the ship's officers appeared on the quay at Jamestown, they were bombarded with questions: "Is Admiral Plampin a married man?" "Has he brought his wife out with him?" With their smirks poorly concealed, they answered "Yes" every time. Let the Admiral sort out his problems for himself!

The Admiral landed alone. Alone he made his way to Plantation House to call upon the Governor. Alone, he made another visit the next day to pay his respects to Lady Lowe and spent more than an hour in her company. On neither visit was any mention made of a Lady Plampin.

Meantime, the lady in question remained on board, thus confirming for the ladies that she was not the Admiral's wife but his mistress – and living openly with him, to boot! Their wrath was well and truly aroused and at their customary gatherings at Plantation House they gave vent to that anger. In their unanimous opinion, the Admiral's conduct was the grossest of insults that could possibly be offered them, considering that he ranked second only to the Governor. What was the world coming to? The Governor must punish him severely. A rumour soon spread from Plantation House – no doubt started with the fervent wish that it might be fulfilled – that the lady would immediately be removed from the island and that the Admiral would be reported and, in all probability, recalled. The rumour quickly reached the Admiral's ears as did the uncompromising sermons of the Reverend Richard Boys, Chaplain to the Honourable East India Company in St Helena. Mr Boys viewed the island as a sink of iniquity, as, indeed, he did the rest of the world. Amongst his duties he had to make the official entries of all births on the island in the parish registers. So it was a righteously indignant Mr Boys who entered the births of the illegitimate children of slave women who had been put in the family way by a prominent islander or senior member of the governor's staff, with the names and titles of the sinning fathers in emphatic script.

When he thought he could nip the immoral behaviour in the bud, he did so with relish in his sermons from the pulpit, and there was no holding back when it came to Admiral Plampin. He beseeched the Admiral to put away from him this accursed woman and to flee the wrath to come while there was yet time. Events were rapidly coming to a head.

Greatly concerned that his plans for a quiet life on St Helena were about to disintegrate in an unwholesome mess, Sir Robert paid another visit to Plantation House and grovelled before Sir Hudson. As Commander-in-Chief of the Naval Station he had every right to independence of action, to do as he wished. But he renounced all his rights and privileges and promised his full cooperation in any measures, however harsh, that the Governor might wish to take against General Bonaparte. In return, he asked only one favour: that he might be allowed to live as he chose. The Governor agreed

Little did the Admiral realize that he could have asked for the moon and been given it. Lowe had got what he wanted all along: authority over the entire island, particularly Longwood and its naval surgeon. He now had access to all the information he wanted about his prisoner – or so he imagined. The British Government had isolated St Helena from the rest of the world, he was intent on isolating Longwood from the rest of the island.

The first apparent consequence of the Governor's agreement was that Mr Boys had to stop preaching against the Admiral and the ladies to cease their malicious gossip. Sir Robert now felt free to bring his mistress ashore and install her at The Briars where he was living with the Balcombes who had yet to leave the island.

And now, would you not expect at least one of the handful of chroniclers who actually saw her to have given their impressions of the lady whose presence was to have such an influence on events?

But no. Balmain's contribution was: "To the great scandal of the colony, he brought a lady with him from London, who, though she uses his name, is only his mistress."

Gourgaud acknowledged her existence.

And, so far as O'Meara was concerned, it was not until two months after her arrival that he made his one and only reference to the affair: In the course of recording some general conversation in his journal, he wrote that Napoleon "blamed Mr. Boys's conduct, for having preached in allusion to the Admiral." And, in a footnote to this, he wrote: "Mr. Boys had thought it a duty to mention something from the pulpit, in censure of an official person, for having set an example of immorality to a small colony, by publicly living with a woman not his wife, and for absenting himself from church."

Both John Stokoe, who had travelled out with the lady, and Betsy Balcombe, who had lived in the same house for the best part of a year are silent about her identity, her age, her appearance, any characteristics she might have possessed and what sort of a life she led on the island.

The fallout from the Admiral's capitulation also affected the naval personnel, for Sir Robert lost no time in publishing a restricting order: "All officers of H.M. Navy, whatever their rank, are strictly forbidden to visit Longwood and its dependencies, or to communicate in any way, by writing or otherwise, under any pretext, with the foreigners detained in the island, without having first presented an explicit and detailed request to the Commander-in-Chief, and obtained his permission." Worthy of his new master!

The officers were mightily upset by this as ever since they knew they were to be posted to St Helena, their dream had been to meet, or at least see, Napoleon. Hitherto, it had been the custom for the resident admiral to present the commanding officer of every newly arrived vessel and, usually, also his senior officers. (Captain Davie had already been presented, with Admiral Plampin before the trouble erupted.) But they knew their dream was dead in the water when the Admiral's secretary told them they were not to be presented as Sir Hudson Lowe did not wish it. What really rubbed salt in the wound was the presentation, by Sir George Bingham, on July 14, of the officers of the 53rd Regiment which was about to leave the island. And then, on September 1, the presentation, again by Sir George, of all thirty-seven officers of the relieving 66th Regiment.

However, the *Conqueror*'s officers weren't short on initiative and set about cultivating O'Meara's acquaintance and besieging him with questions. He dined several times on board the *Conqueror* and, as his hosts had anticipated, invited them in return to visit him at Longwood. The Admiral sometimes granted them the necessary passes.

Although aware that something unusual was afoot, O'Meara gave no indication of understanding *why*. He sensed that the Governor's attitude towards him was undergoing a none-too-subtle change as he was being asked more and more questions about the nature of Napoleon's conversations and what he had been saying about himself (Lowe). The Governor also, in the course of a long conversation, "part of it not of a very agreeable nature" said he did not consider O'Meara had been doing sufficient to undeceive General Bonaparte who was "so much in the *dark* respecting *his* (Lowe's) character." O'Meara, by and large, only reported Napoleon's observations on events when Napoleon told him he might, and even then he would water down the comments about the Governor.

The first critical moment, so far as O'Meara was concerned, arrived on July 24, when he was subjected to an interrogation by the Governor in front of Sir Thomas Reade and Major Gorrequer. During this Lowe became extremely angry simply because O'Meara's opinions differed from his own.

It suddenly dawned on O'Meara that times had changed since Admiral Malcolm was now no longer there to hold the balance between Governor and General. Any hope of these two seeing eye to eye had vanished. Instead, Lowe was treating O'Meara as a surrogate Napoleon and holding him responsible for everthing the real Napoleon did and said. That made O'Meara the butt for all the Governor's ill-temper.

O'Meara came away from the meeting determined that any hope of a quiet life lay in sticking as much as possible to his medical duties, and to avoid all unnecessary communication with a man (Lowe) who could use his authority to take advantage of a junior officer (O'Meara) in such a despicable manner. Some hope!

A second critical moment made its appearance on August 14. O'Meara had gone on a routine visit to Plantation House. No sooner was he across the doorstep than Lowe raised the subject of the Amherst Mission, in particular what Napoleon had said to Lord Amherst about his ill-treatment – a topic still rankling merrily along six weeks after his lordship had left the island. When Lowe asked O'Meara to reprise the conversation, O'Meara saw what was going to happen but didn't feel authorized to refuse as Napoleon had told him he was free to repeat these remarks to the Governor:

"Neither your prince nor both your houses of parliament can oblige me to see *mon geolier et mon bourreau. Ce n'est pas l'habit qui fait le geolier, c'est la manière et les moeurs.*" ("…my jailer and my executioner. It is not the clothes that make the jailer, it is the manners and the moral integrity.")Furious, Lowe asked why the General had used such an expression. O'Meara answered that that was something he couldn't possibly know. The Governor then proceeded to unleash his anger on O'Meara, ending with:

"You are not authorized by me, Sir, to communicate with General Bonaparte on any other than medical subjects; and if you hold any others with him, it is at your own peril, unless you make such communications known to me, and thereby free yourself from the responsibility. Your business is not to act from your own judgment or discretion, but to ask what you may be permitted to do." This certainly was telling him, but it was like water off a duck's back for all the effect it had on O'Meara.

The next time he visited Plantation House, O'Meara had to endure another interrogation that was almost a repeat of the one the previous week. At the end of it he told the Governor that he was quite mistaken if he expected him to report on his conversations with Napoleon.

Throughout August Napoleon continued in good spirits, cracking jokes and taking more exercise. However, coinciding with some exceptionally wet days in the first week of September, he began complaining of minor, short-lived ailments which he attributed, and with reason, to the damp chill of Longwood. He kept the fires burning in the four rooms he himself used but, as he couldn't abide the smell of burning coal, the supply of wood was in danger of running out. Whereupon the familiar round of exchanges sparked off by shortages began again. Cipriani prevailed upon Captain Henry Blakeney, the new orderly officer from the 66th, to write to the purveyors asking them for thirty hundredweight of wood which they would pay for themselves. However, as the Governor's allowance was no more than three hundredweight daily, O'Meara was ordered to Plantation House to account for the situation.

"There are far too many fires at Longwood," accused the Governor (there were twenty-three), "they have no business with so many."

"But," answered O'Meara, "the ladies and children need fires burning all the time because Longwood is so damp."

"Lady Lowe has no fire in *her* room," countered the Governor. A stupid remark, if ever there was one since the conditions in the two houses were such, as O'Meara pointed out, that any sort of comparison was impossible. He went on to suggest that, as Napoleon could not bear the smell of coal, his allocation might be sent to the soldiers' camp in exchange for wood.

"I do not like to humour any person's whims," was the response.

The next day the Governor told O'Meara to talk the matter over with Montholon whose clothes and those of his wife had been ruined by the damp, in spite of their fires. O'Meara told him that the Governor had decided on the amount of fuel to be sent to Longwood by allowing twice as much coal as used at Plantation House plus three hundredweight of wood daily. He would have increased these amounts had any application been made, but Montholon had made none. The reason, Montholon explained, was the worry that he might be slighted or refused.

However, a day or two later Montholon did ask both O'Meara and Blakeney to inspect his apartments. O'Meara concluded: "The rooms, especially the Countess's bedroom, the children's room, and bath room, were certainly in a shocking state, from the extreme humidity of the place. The walls were covered with green fur and mould; damp and cold to the touch, notwithstanding the fires which were constantly kept in them. I never saw a human habitation in a more mouldy or humid state, in which opinion the orderly officer agreed." For all the good it would do, the allowance was increased.

O'Meara was in trouble again at the autumn meeting of the Deadwood races. The Governor had found out that he had borrowed a couple of Napoleon's horses, one for Betsy Balcombe and the other for Stokoe. During an interval Lowe sent for him and proceeded to berate him with such vigour that his gestures attracted the attention of other spectators. To have dared to lend any of General Bonaparte's horses without his (the Governor's) permission was the "greatest piece of presumption he had ever witnessed."

"To think that I have had to come to St Helena," O'Meara counter-attacked, "to learn that it is a crime to borrow a horse for the use of a young lady." However, he knew this attack on him was only yet another pretext for Lowe to vent his anger on a surrogate Napoleon. Every week, horses were sent down to Jamestown for Dr Livingstone and others to ride up to Longwood, without there ever having been the slightest hint that it was necessary to apply to the Governor for permission. Moreover, General Gourgaud had directed that a horse should always be in the stables at O'Meara's command.

The real Napoleon, meanwhile, had again been enjoying a day at the races from an upstairs window in the Bertrand house.

A week later, O'Meara was summoned to Plantation House and told to bring a report on General Bonaparte's state of health. This he did because there was nothing of significance to report.

The Governor then informed him that others had also been reporting on the General's health. Thus, Madame Bertrand had told the Commissioners, when they met after the races, that he was extremely unwell and just because he may have been seen standing on the veranda did not mean he was in good health.

Fanny Bertrand must have had the second sight because the next day Napoleon again showed evidence of scurvy. He had not slept at all well and when O'Meara saw him, in his bath, he was feeling low and complaining of toothache. His gums were once again spongy and bled at the slightest touch. His appetite was poor and from time to time he felt nauseous. His ankles and legs were swollen. As exercise was, by mutual consent, out of the question, all O'Meara could do was recommend antiscorbutic vegetables and suggest he took a dose of physic (unspecified) but Napoleon objected because, "Take a dose of medicine once and in all probability you will be obliged to take an additional hundred afterwards" – an oft-echoed sentiment to this day. He then had his breakfast of two or three radishes, a little toast and butter, followed by a small *café au lait*. Not exactly in tune with his doctor's recommendations.

Things did not improve over the next two days and, in view of the importance of his patient and the peculiar attitude of the Governor towards himself, O'Meara considered it prudent to call in a second opinion but when he suggested Baxter, Napoleon would have none of it:

"There is no need for it. If all the colleges of medicine in France and England were assembled, they would give the same advice as you have done – take exercise on horseback. I myself know as well as any physician what is necessary for me. It is exercise. Calling in Baxter to me would be like sending a physician to a man who was starving with hunger, instead of giving him a loaf of bread. I have no objection to your letting him know my state of health if you like, and I am well aware that he will say *exercise*....

"Until matters are put on a similar footing to what they were in Cockburn's time – and they had the approval of the British Government – I shall never stir out." Remember Cockburn's prophetic words? "The Bonaparte Detention Bill is positive in its instructions; no changes should have been made, except such as were ordered by the Prince Regent and the Privy Council, and signed by the Regent or Lord Liverpool; not by Lord Bathurst. I consider all restrictions not made by them as null. . . . To avoid the possibility of being insulted, I have shut myself up. . . . By prohibiting me to speak to people I might meet, he offered me the greatest insult which could be offered to man.

"Lord Bathurst's intentions are to impose restrictions of such a nature," once he got going there was no stopping the flood, "that unless I am to become an object of contempt in the eyes of the world, I must imprison myself. Thus, in the course of time, bringing on disease which, in a body impaired by confinement and with blood thinned, must prove mortal." [Is it even remotely on the cards that Napoleon suspected he was anaemic? The possibility that he had iron-deficiency anaemia does, however, crop up in three years time.] "I may thus expire in protracted agonies which give the appearance of a natural death. This is the plan, and is a manner of assassination just as certain, but more cruel and criminal, than the sword or the pistol." The prophet is without honour in his isle of exile!

Not long afterwards the Governor came to Longwood and having enquired about the General's health asked what he and O'Meara had been talking about. O'Meara thereupon obliged, omitting the insults. When he arrived at a mention of the Amherst affair, Lowe pricked up his ears and called in Gorrequer as witness. Lowe was still desperately concerned with what Napoleon might have said to Lord Amherst and thus what Lord Amherst might have passed on to Lord Bathurst. He continued worrying away at it as if repeated questioning might somehow reveal a truth that accorded with his wishes. Getting nothing out of O'Meara, Lowe launched into one of his harangues accusing him of being of the same way of thinking as the General. It finally ended with a threat to remove him from the island.

"I should immediately and without awaiting the orders of Government send you off the island, Sir. I have received no official intelligence from Government concerning your appointment; you are not of my choosing; you are only permitted to visit General Bonaparte as a medical man."

Quite a revelation and no mistake. Could Lowe *really* have believed that O'Meara was just a supernumerary surgeon on board the *Northumberland* who had found himself deputed to look after Napoleon with no governmental authority to do so (despite the evidence of his description on the bills for his pay)? Could the Government have failed to tell him that O'Meara had been officially appointed as Napoleon's surgeon and that his choosing had nothing to do with it? Or had the "official intelligence" been conveniently 'lost in the post'? For the moment I propose leaving these questions hanging in the air.

By the end of September, Napoleon was in much better spirits, doubtless because he was feeling better. He had been eating vegetables with enthusiasm and benefit, his gums were improving and, though his legs were just as swollen, they were not so painful. O'Meara could find nothing seriously wrong, but he did wonder about the imperial legs.

Shortly after, Lowe called on Bertrand who told him that Napoleon was really in a much worse state of health than O'Meara had made out. O wretched Governor! How can you know who or what to believe?

* * *

And now, *mon ami(e)*, you understand how it was that the mere presence on the island of the Admiral's mistress could have such disastrous consequences. Admiral Plampin had sold his soul to the devil in return for a quiet life in her arms. In the first two months the effects were felt mainly by those concerned with Napoleon's welfare, with relations between Governor and General reduced to an unpleasant slanging match and O'Meara, the constant go-between, left wondering why on earth the Governor should be taking it out on him with such venom. You are beginning to see clearly what poor O'Meara was up against. And the man who should have shielded him from these assaults was, in fact, the cause of them and completely under the Governor's thumb.

~14~ *John Stokoe's instinct for survival lets him down*

(OCTOBER, 1817)

The first day of October, 1817, brought with it the first signs of the diseases that were to be with Napoleon for the rest of his life. Thus far there had only been a gradual decline in his health due to the generally unhealthy conditions at Longwood, his lack of exercise and the governor's unrelenting persecution, but nothing that couldn't be remedied.

When O'Meara visited Napoleon at 8am on that day, he found him complaining of a dull pain in his right side under the ribs which he had first experienced the previous morning, added to which he had a numb sensation in his right shoulder. He also was aware of a lump in his right side which, he said, he had never felt before. O'Meara reckoned it was due to costiveness – well, you do don't you when you know the patient is chronically constipated? The signs of scurvy were unchanged and his pulse rate was 68 per minute (which, in his case, may be regarded as raised by about ten beats per minute, indicating that something of an inflammatory or infective nature was possibly going on). Should the symptoms get worse or new ones appear, O'Meara was prepared to change the diagnosis to hepatitis, otherwise he was sticking to constipation. Napoleon then took a salt-water bath during which he conducted a long conversation on medical matters.

Over the next twenty-four hours his legs swelled up a little more, he slept badly and ate scarcely anything. The bath had brought relief, but there was no more water available.

On the third, O'Meara found that Napoleon's right side felt firmer than the left. There was also a visible swelling which was painful when he pressed hard. Napoleon admitted that he had first noticed it about two months previously but had attributed it to obesity. Now, though, he wondered whether it might have something to do with an enlarged liver. O'Meara recommended calomel (mercurous chloride, a purgative) and all the usual treatments – though I doubt whether Napoleon actually took the calomel. O'Meara also continued to urge the need for exercise, making the point that he was bound, as his medical adviser, to do his best to get him to use *any* remedy that might be beneficial. He then, once again, asked his permission to call in Baxter. Napoleon said he would consider it should the symptoms worsen, but only if the Governor didn't try to interfere – if he did, never!

When O'Meara presented his medical report to the Governor, he was told it was too detailed and he must prepare another that could be made public – in other words, one that made no specific reference to liver disease as this could put the British in bad odour for detaining the General on an unhealthy island. He was having none of this – let the Governor fillet the report for himself.

* * *

O'Meara and Stokoe were idly strolling in the Longwood garden when Napoleon came out through the billiard-room door accompanied by the Montholons. He sat himself down on the steps with Madame beside him. When he saw the two surgeons, Montholon came across to ask who Stokoe was. After a quick word with Napoleon he came back to say that the Emperor would be glad to meet him.

"Surgeon *Conqueror*, man-of-war. Fine ship," said the Emperor before, much to everyone's relief, O'Meara told him that Stokoe spoke Italian.

"Whereabouts have you been in Italy?"

"Gaeta was the only place where I landed, but I spent about three years in the Mediterranean, most of the time in Sicily."

"Ah! a beautiful island, a little better than this one! Are you senior to O'Meara?"

"Yes , Sir, by ten years."

"Then you can command him?" Not sure where this might be leading, Stokoe avoided giving an answer.

"What service have you seen?"

"I was surgeon of a 74 [the *Thunderer*] in the battle of Trafalgar, and in the passage of the Dardanelles."

"What countryman are you?"

"From the north of England."

"That is a mountainous country, is it not?"

"It is."

Napoleon continued questioning Stokoe about this and that, quite charming him in the process. This effect became all too evident when they got back to O'Meara's quarters.

"Beforehand I had a clear picture in my mind of the man I expected to see," Stokoe began, " but he was so totally the opposite that we hadn't been talking for more than two minutes before I felt myself as much at ease as if I'd been speaking to an equal. I'm not ashamed to admit I felt so well disposed towards him, that I could have been his ambassador to Sir Hudson, and gone at that very moment to beg him to remove all those restrictions that made the General refuse to take exercise."

The next morning, Stokoe felt duty bound to call at The Briars to report his visit to the Admiral even though he had had a permit to visit O'Meara and the meeting with Napoleon had been accidental and impossible to avoid. The Admiral thought differently; Stokoe was roundly ticked off and told it was unnecessary to be polite to the General. The Admiral's lady was in the room throughout the reprimand and at its end asked Stokoe what he thought of Napoleon. He said his opinion had completely changed since he had met the man, to which 'Lady' Plampin responded that Napoleon must be an extraordinary man, for almost every stranger who approached him came away with the same favourable opinion. And nothing more shall we learn about this femme fatale's views on life, on people, on anything.

Immediately he had finished with Stokoe, the Admiral wrote to Captain Davie with an order that whenever any officer of the squadron was invited to dine with either O'Meara or the orderly officer at Longwood, they were not to communicate in any way whatsoever with the General, even if he should ask them to do so, unless he (Plampin) had given them permission.

But Stokoe's troubles were only just beginning. Not having reported to Plantation House of his own accord, he was summoned there by the Governor who feigned surprise that he had not seen him sooner. Stokoe said he had called on the Admiral and given him details of all that had transpired; but he would gladly repeat them if the Governor felt it was that important – he had nothing to hide. What he had overlooked was the first principle of an unmolested life on the island, namely, anything concerning General Bonaparte, however small or insignificant, was to be reported to Sir Hudson, in person and preferably without delay.

"In what language was the conversation held?" asked the Governor.

"In Italian."

The look that distorted Lowe's face made Stokoe fear he was in considerable pain until he realized the man was staring directly at him. His fluency in Italian meant he had been able to converse freely with Napoleon and when he mentioned he had served three years in Sicily, the Governor's discomfiture was complete. Those years would have coincided with the time that Lowe had commanded at Capri – Stokoe would thus be aware of the reputation he had acquired when he surrendered an allegedly impregnable island to an allegedly numerically inferior force. Stokoe left the interview feeling only contempt for the Governor, as he believed he now had confirmation that the low opinion in which Lowe had been held at Palermo was thoroughly justified.

Stokoe knew that Napoleon had refused to see Baxter because of the Governor's hand in the matter. However, when the Admiral gave him a note from O'Meara saying that Napoleon was quite prepared to see him instead because he had made such a good impression, Stokoe begged the Admiral to let him refuse. This uncharacteristic response was prompted by his instinct for survival. He knew the Governor did not trust O'Meara's recent reports on Napoleon's declining state of health. Consequently, if he visited Napoleon alone with O'Meara and agree with his diagnosis, the Governor would accuse him of being influenced by his friend. At the least, this would draw unfavourable attention to himself.

The Admiral told Stokoe he was free to act as he felt fit, but any consequences of his actions would be on his own head. Stokoe therefore decided to use the Admiral's pass to go to Longwood to explain his refusal and get O'Meara's opinion. This he did, but his friend could not persuade him to change his mind. Little did he expect to find he had only exchanged the frying pan of Plampin for the fire of Lowe.

A week later Stokoe was told to present himself in Reade's office in the Castle. The Governor appeared from the next room and, taking some papers from his pocket, said he couldn't convince the people at Longwood that he had nothing to do with Stokoe's refusal to see General Bonaparte. "I wish you to tell me why you refused."

This was a nasty one as he obviously couldn't give the true reason; instead he went half way by saying he was very unwilling to go to Longwood, but if compelled to visit General Bonaparte he would naturally, with a patient of such importance, wish to do so in company with other medical men to have the benefit of their opinions. This seemed to satisfy the Governor who told him to write a letter to the Admiral stating these facts. "Let me see it before you send it."

Stokoe's letter simply repeated his explanation, but the Governor didn't approve and began writing himself. The main difference came with the last line, "…he would wish to visit the General with other medical men, excluding his private attendant."

Whatever the consequences Stokoe was not prepared to let that pass; it would give the impression that he was unwilling to consult with O'Meara, which was far from being the case. The Governor changed the wording to "…in addition to his private attendant." Then, after a minute or two he pushed the paper away and, throwing his pen down violently, left the room in a towering rage, "You can send your letter, Sir."

Since Lowe was trying to engineer O'Meara's recall, Stokoe's signature on his first revision of the letter would have been invaluable: it would have enabled him to write to Lord Bathurst with proof that, if the surgeon of the flagship refused to consult with him, O'Meara was clearly of undesirable character. Oh! Sir Hudson, is there no end to your deviousness?

* * *

And now, *mon ami(e)* you understand why Stokoe was having such a terrible time at the hands of the Governor. He realized the peril he faced but could do nothing to avoid it.

~15~
Paranoia in Plantation House

(OCTOBER – DECEMBER, 1817)

Napoleon had been restless on the night of the tenth of October and in the morning the pain in his right side and shoulder was worse and his appetite poor. He also had a return of what he called the palpitations (a symptom he hadn't mentioned before and which he attributed to having sat too long in the sun – but it was to receive a non-medical importance all its own). Later in the day he had a hot bath to ease his pains.

From the fourteenth to the end of the month, the question of what Napoleon should be called in O'Meara's bulletins, and who should see them, shuttled back and forth between O'Meara and Plantation House. It all began when Montholon and Gourgaud were asked by someone in the street how Napoleon's palpitations were. Neither Frenchman knew that he had been afflicted in this way, but their questioner had been informed by the various bulletins sent to the Governor. Although Napoleon came to hear about the breach of confidentiality, that certainly wasn't the aspect that bothered him most. He had asked O'Meara to show him one of his own bulletins. Glancing through it he noticed that O'Meara had referred to him as 'General'.

"I shall never consent to be so styled by you or by any other person acting as my physician. As such you must possess a certain share of my confidence, without which you could not be acquainted with my symptoms. A physician is to the body what a confessor is to the soul and is bound to keep such confession equally sacred, unless permitted to divulge it. In future you shall show me all your reports on my health before sending them to the Governor."

However, of even greater concern to Napoleon was the fact that the bulletins were given to the Commissioners for onward transmission to their courts. For these people to see his personal physician refer to him, not as 'Emperor' but as mere 'General' would amount to acquiescence on his part to such a title – something he would rather die than consent to. If O'Meara did not agree with this, Napoleon would never again consult him as his physician.

O'Meara sighed a sigh. They had been all over this from a different angle just a year before, but could they hope that some sort of a settlement might be reached this year? No! O'Meara knew the Governor would never allow him, or any one else for that matter, to style Napoleon '*l'Empereur*' (he couldn't stop Montholon, though) and so suggested 'Napoleon' or 'Napoleon Bonaparte' but Napoleon refused. He didn't care, he said, if, in his verbal reports, O'Meara called him '*generale*', '*boja*' or '*tiranno Bonaparte*', but in the written reports, it was '*l'Empereur*'.

The Governor did not allow it. He was willing to accept 'Napoleon Bonaparte' even though he knew it would not move matters forward. He also saw no objection "for the time being" to Napoleon seeing the reports before he did; however, it was a matter he could give no definite ruling on as it required consideration.

An acceptable escape route would have been the use of an incognito but, as Napoleon feelingly recollected, the British Government had given no answer to his previous proposal. It would now be the height of insult to insist on naming him as they liked. The more they endeavoured to humiliate him the more firmly would he grasp his title.

O'Meara's next suggestion was to use the word 'personage' with which Napoleon agreed though he preferred 'patient' ('*le malade*'), again provided the reports were shown to him first. Need it be said that the Governor rejected this solution?

One unattractive upshot of an unattractive argument was that Napoleon would no longer consult his physician about his complaints and would answer no relevant questions. In fact, were it not for the confidence he had in him, Napoleon would have dispensed with his services completely the moment he had learned that O'Meara went regularly to Plantation House every Tuesday and Saturday, by order of the Governor.

"You may tell him," said Napoleon after O'Meara had tried in vain to extract some medical information, "that I conceive his object to be to deprive me of all medical aid, and by that to arrive sooner at the end which he proposes. I do not esteem life so much as to allow my physician to be made a spy. Tell him that I said his views are directed to lessening the confidence I had in you, and to make you a spy, or to make me suspect that you are."

O'Meara passed part of this conversation on to the Governor who, hesitatingly, said he would demand no more bulletins unless Napoleon knew he had asked for them.

Napoleon responded favourably to this and brought O'Meara up-to-date with his symptoms. He was, he said, never free from a dull pain or an uneasy sensation in his right side; his legs continued to swell; he suffered occasionally from nausea and was seriously short of sleep. Since his appetite was still poor he had decided that, in future, he would have only one regular meal a day and that at two or three o'clock. To O'Meara's consternation, this might put him in danger of becoming malnourished since, for some time, he had been eating very little.

Napoleon then asked him whether another person, or a witness as he called him, was present at his twice weekly conversations with the Governor and when O'Meara confirmed that this was so, he said:

"Then, doctor, you will be made to say what he wishes you to say. It would not surprise me to learn that he had a report of what you said already prepared before you even arrive there. This will be produced against you in the future. It places you in a very dangerous situation." More often than not, the witness was his secretary, Gorrequer, for whom the conversion of what was said into what the Governor wanted to have been said, came as second nature.

O'Meara's visits to Plantation House were getting more and more unpleasant but he persisted in his refusal to divulge the content of Napoleon's conversations. This always brought the Governor to boiling point and on one occasion he shouted that he conceived him to be a jackal running about in search of news for General Bonaparte. O'Meara replied that he would not be a jackal, or a spy, or an informer for him or for anyone else.

"What do you mean, Sir," said he, "by a spy or an informer?"

"If I comply with your directions to inform you of the conversations I have with Napoleon, I should regard myself as both."

"You are to consider yourself," he was in a paroxysm of rage, "as forbidden to have any communication whatsoever with Napoleon Bonaparte except upon medical subjects." Surely Lowe could not have forgotten that such a ban was already in force? But just in case, O'Meara asked for it to be put in writing. The Governor refused.

When he had calmed down, Lowe told O'Meara he would no longer be required twice a week at Plantation House. Instead, he expected him to confer every week with Mr Baxter on the state of Napoleon's health – hoping thereby to get a reasonably accurate account of Napoleon's well-being or otherwise. O'Meara agreed to this as Napoleon had no objections to verbal discussions. He was also heartily glad that he was no longer required to put in an appearance at Plantation House.

On the twenty-fifth O'Meara managed to burrow deep under the Governor's skin by yet again refusing to divulge his conversations with Napoleon. "It is a duty, Sir, you owe to the

British Government." O'Meara answered, as before, that it would be acting the part of a spy, an informer, and this time he added a *mouton*.

Lowe said nothing for a few moments, then "What is the meaning of the word *mouton*?"

"*Mouton* means a person who insinuates himself into the confidence of another, for the purpose of betraying it."

When this had sunk in, the Governor burst into a veritable paroxysm of fury: O'Meara had just insulted him in his official capacity in the grossest way possible, no one who used such language would be permitted to sit in his presence. O'Meara was ordered to leave the room, at which he calmly drew the Governor's attention to the fact that he hadn't come voluntarily and, in any event, he entered the house only when compelled to do so.

"Leave the room, Sir! Leave the room!" which he continued bawling out after the order had been well and truly obeyed.

Into December, and on the seventh O'Meara was able to tell Baxter that he had at last persuaded Napoleon to take some medicine (he didn't say what) which he had administered himself (which meant that Napoleon had actually taken it). Whatever it was, it had been only of temporary benefit.

On the ninth O'Meara received a signal to go to Plantation House where the Governor, looking serious, said he wanted to speak to him on a non-medical matter. Was it true, he asked, that he was a medium for communication between the French at Longwood and the islanders? And he was not meaning communications to favour General Bonaparte's escape from the island.

"If going to the shops and buying articles for Countess Bertrand and Countess Montholon, or anyone else at Longwood, could be construed as carrying on communications or correspondence for them, I must certainly plead guilty."

"Have you written to a person in the town asking them to send up some articles for Madame Bertrand?" The Governor's spy network was indeed working overtime.

"Certainly, I have written to Mr Darling [the works foreman] to send up some basins, chamber utensils and other household articles."

"That was a breach of orders. You have been forbidden to be the bearer of any message or communication not medical. What business had you to do so? If Madame Bertrand wants anything of the kind, let her apply to the orderly officer. Why hadn't she done so?"

"In the first place, cleanliness is necessary to prevent sickness and so everything relating to it is medical. In the second place, the orderly officer was not at Longwood when Madame Bertrand asked me; and had he been, delicacy would prevent a lady from making demands to him for certain necessary articles which she could with propriety mention to her surgeon. I do not conceive it to be a crime to ask a tradesman to purchase chamber utensils, or similar articles, either for Madame Bertrand or myself."

As usual, Lowe flew into a violent passion. "I will not allow you to insult me in my capacity of governor. How dare you order articles to be sent out of the king's stores without consulting me? Or having them charged to those stores?"

"I said nothing about having them charged to the king's stores."

O'Meara again asked for written orders and was again refused.

On his next visit to Plantation House which was by order of the Governor himself, he was questioned about his appointment as surgeon to Napoleon. Lowe's line of attack was that he was not the General's surgeon but merely tolerated to visit him. And this despite the evidence of the bills that O'Meara drew for his pay on the Navy Board which Lowe well knew were worded "as surgeon to Napoleon Bonaparte and suite." The "official intelligence" had undoubtedly been "lost in the post"!

Lowe then changed tack and asked whether he regarded himself as independent of him. O'Meara told Lowe he could best answer that himself as he should know the extent of his authority. After strutting about the room for a while exclaiming against O'Meara's conduct and with a terrible expression on his face, the Governor unleashed his fury:

"This is my office, Sir, and there is the door leading to it. When I send for you on duty, you will come in at that door; but do not put your foot in any other part of my house, or come in at any other entrance."

"It is not for my own pleasure, or by my own desire that I ever set foot in any part of this house." And O'Meara made his escape.

It now seems scarcely credible, but on O'Meara's next two visits to that house he was to be interrogated, yet again, about Napoleon and the visit of Lord Amherst. However, on these occasions Lowe was more concerned with Napoleon's insults than with the conditions of his captivity. In particular he wanted to know whether O'Meara had been given the authority to repeat the insults. This was regardless of the fact that O'Meara had been through an almost verbatim examination on the fourteenth of August but, as he guessed, Lowe was still desperately looking for answers that best suited whatever purposes he now had in mind. The Governor's paranoid personality was showing every sign of tipping over into a full-blown psychoneurotic disorder.

Further evidence of this came on the thirteenth when the Governor produced a copy of the *Morning Chronicle* of the previous September containing a detail of a conversation between Napoleon and "some English gentleman" which thoroughly upset him. Because of the context, he had come to the conclusion that the gentleman was either O'Meara or Admiral Malcolm. When O'Meara convincingly denied being the gentleman, Lowe was most anxious that he should help him saddle the Admiral with the blame, but O'Meara was having none of it. Indeed, he saw at once from the context that the gentleman must have been Sir Henry Ellis, the secretary to the Amherst Mission! Nevertheless, he was only partly right: Ellis had not written the offending passage himself but had had its insertion imposed on him by one of Lord Bathurst's deputies.

The twentieth brought yet another aggressive interview at Plantation House, starting with a series of questions about how General Bonaparte spent his time.

"I cannot tell, Sir."

"Yes, you can, Sir. You well know what he does there; you do not do your duty to Government."

Getting no response, the Governor stomped around the room, stopping occasionally to glare and shout at O'Meara who occupied himself by taking out his watch and timing the exhibition – he more than once thought he was about to be assaulted. At length Lowe launched into another series of interrogations, this time seeking the name of the person who, a year before, had told O'Meara that Lord Liverpool had intervened and prevented his (O'Meara's) removal from the island. O'Meara refused and after enduring progressively more violent abuse, he said:

"As my replies only bring upon me abuse, bad language and bad treatment, I must decline to give you any more answers on the subject."

"Put down, Major Gorrequer, that Mr O'Meara refuses to answer."

O'Meara was then subjected to another long and abusive harangue about his improper conduct because of his refusal to implicate Admiral Malcolm in the newspaper article. Could Sir Hudson Lowe let nothing rest?

O'Meara was permitted to depart.

* * *

In case you might think that I am being unduly harsh on the poor man in my telling of the behaviour and actions of Sir Hudson

Lowe, the *military* governor, you should not forget that he was also the *civil* governor and, as such, accountable to the Honourable East India Company. As military governor, he was answerable to the British Government and thus, particularly with Napoleon in his care, enmeshed in the treacherous web of politics. As civil governor, he administered the civil affairs of St Helena and politics was no part of the relationship between himself and the Company. You might, therefore, reasonably expect the correspondence between these two parties to provide a balanced and unbiased insight into Lowe's personality.

Mr Thomas Breame, manager of the Company's farms, had been under suspicion for about a year of feathering his own nest by selling stock and failing to account for money received, and by committing a number of other financial misdemeanours. An island council meeting on December 8, 1817, decided that, as he had been unable to give a plausible account of what had been going on, they would set up an enquiry "to ascertain any loss which the Company may have sustained whilst the farms were under his management, and whether they are of such a nature as to justify any further proceedings against him."

Without waiting for the outcome of the enquiry – which proved to be long, complicated and inconclusive – Lowe immediately removed him from the management of the farms.

Although this event was the burden of the exasperated Company Directors' letter of May 2, 1820, it was by no means the only occasion on which the Governor had incurred their displeasure.

In the early days of his governorship, the correspondence between Lowe and the Directors had been business-like, but gradually Lowe became intolerant of what he saw as criticism of his administration of civil affairs. In the letter of May 2 – an exquisite example of convoluted, circumlocutory writing – the Directors set out their dissatisfaction, not only with the manner in which he had conducted their affairs, but also with the tone which he, their servant, had seen fit to adopt in reporting to them.

After admonishing Secret and Confidential the letter began: "In the perusal of the letters from St. Helena dated in the last year, it has been impossible for us to pass unnoticed the Tone and Stile in which you have been betrayed not only in the Letters coming immediately from yourself but occasionally also in the Despatches from the Governor and Council.

"Although we are persuaded that you were not influenced by intentional disrespect to the Court in what we have here alluded to, we are confident that on deliberately reflecting upon the exceptionable matters which we are about to point out you will acknowledge that they are liable to such construction, and will not fail to admit their impropriety considering the relative situation in which you stand to the Court.

"You appear to entertain an Idea that because, in the exercise of that authority which we possess by legislative enactments, we have differed from you in opinion upon some parts of your Proceedings, we have therefore withheld or withdrawn Our support from your Government, but this conclusion is by no means warranted by the orders we have given on certain points when they happened to be in opposition to the views you may have taken, and a moment's attention must convince you that if we were to abstain from controlling and setting aside any Act of our Governments abroad on account of the mistaken construction which may be given to our Orders, there is at once an end of our Authority and the situation of the Governors and Governed would virtually be removed.

"We can find nothing in reperusal of our orders of 22nd December 1819, upon the subject of Mr Breame's removal from the management of the Company's Farms, which will justify the frequent repetition in your Letter of the 30th March 1820 of the words Censure and Reproach applied to them. It is true, we expressed disapprobation of your Proceedings, but certainly not in terms liable to such a construction …"

After referring to other instances when Lowe had upset the Directors and taken exception to their reprimands, the letter continued: "We cannot suffer Ourselves to be thus dictated to as to the manner in which we may chuse to seek for information relative to our affairs at St. Helena, or the Persons to whom we may see proper to apply …"

Then, having drawn attention to other parts of Lowe's letter that "appeared exceptionable" to them, the Directors proceeded "to notice some passages in the Letter from the Governor and Council which are equally so." This they did in detail before concluding:

"We shall pursue the subject no further. Enough has been said, we trust, to convince you, Sir, upon a calm and dispassionate review of all the circumstances to which we have called your attention, that the view you have taken of Our Orders is not warranted by any fair construction of them, and that the Tone and Temper in which you have indulged in discussing them are as unsuitable to the relative situation in which you stand towards the Court, as they would be incompatible with a due regard to the authority we possess, were we to suffer them to pass without animadversion. We cannot suppose that you have intentionally shewn Disrespect to that Authority in the several instances which we have pointed out, and if (as we cannot for a moment allow ourselves to doubt) you shall on mature reflection be convinced that you have been led into Error or Misconception, we would gladly hope, that this unpleasant Correspondence will here terminate.

"We are Sir, Your loving Friends".

This masterpiece of a reprimand was signed by thirteen directors who could stand in judgment of Lowe as their servant, the civil governor of St Helena. How he acted as military governor was no concern of theirs. Evidently, though, he was the same paranoid governor in both roles.

* * *

And now, *mon ami*(*e*), you will appreciate that Napoleon was beginning to show signs of something wrong in his abdomen. The Governor believed he had O'Meara at his beck and call. O'Meara still imagined he was answerable only to the Admiral and still could not understand why the Governor was treating him so badly. Napoleon was becoming more and more cagey about who had access to O'Meara's medical bulletins. Lowe's behaviour as both military and civil governor indicated beyond doubt that he was paranoid. All in all, things were not looking good for Napoleon's medical management. The bizarre effects of 'Lady' Plampin's presence on the island knew no bounds.

~16~
This little piggy-in-the-middle is sent all the way home

(FEBRUARY – JULY, 1818)

For a week or two at the beginning of 1818, O'Meara's reports on Napoleon's health were brief and in the nature of "much the same" or "indisposition has rather increased". Naturally, the Governor was dissatisfied with this and thought he saw a way of extracting more information from O'Meara. He called him to Plantation House and told him he had heard in an "indirect manner" that General Bonaparte was in a much worse state of health than indicated by his reports. So, to save him having to come to Plantation House every day he had a report to make, he should make them verbally to Mr Baxter or Sir Thomas Reade whenever he went to town – as he had done previously. This suited O'Meara's book since, as I have mentioned, Napoleon had authorized verbal communications. To set the ball rolling the Governor told him there and then to give a report to Major Gorrequer who was, as always, on the spot to record Lowe's conversations.

O'Meara obliged: Napoleon's headaches were occurring less frequently; he did, however, have symptoms of dyspepsia, notably nausea and flatulence, and his bowels were very costive. The general state of his health was showing no signs of improvement and the pain in his side and the swelling of his legs were unchanged. Before he left, O'Meara asked if he might have a small still, or alembic, so that he could make some orange-flower water of which there was none to be had on the island. This would have been of considerable comfort to Napoleon but, despite asking repeatedly, the request always fell on deaf ears.

On February 17, O'Meara was summoned to Plantation House to be roundly abused on a number of counts. The Governor began by asking whether he had shown Captain Blakeney the letter mentioning Lord Liverpool's intervention to prevent his (O'Meara's) removal from the island.

"No," said O'Meara, "because you had left the decision to me. At the time I did offer to show it to him but you refused; you said you considered the offer to be an insult." Lowe then told O'Meara to show the letter to Blakeney but, not knowing why the Governor had changed his mind, he declined feeling he was on delicate ground. This did not please Lowe one little bit. Lowe next accused O'Meara of constantly insulting him as Governor. O'Meara apologized if such constructions, so foreign to his intentions, should have been put on his words. The Governor, who didn't appreciate the sarcasm, rose to his feet and, glaring menacingly at O'Meara, changed direction:

"Upon your word of honour, Sir, I ask if you have had any conversations with Napoleon Bonaparte, other than on medical subjects, in the past month?"

"Perhaps there may have been, but of no interest." O'Meara certainly knew how to wind the Governor up!

"I do not allow *you*, Sir, to be a judge of whether they were uninteresting or otherwise. You have no authority for holding *any* communication with Napoleon Bonaparte, unless upon medical subjects, and then only when sent for to attend to him." Lowe had just inserted yet another restriction, whether intentionally or not but it would have been recorded by Gorrequer: He was now permitting O'Meara to visit Napoleon "only when sent for".

"Have you had any communication with any other person of his suite?"

"Certainly, Sir, I have had."

Without waiting to learn whether these were medical or

otherwise, the Governor burst out:

"You have no authority, Sir, to hold any communication whatsoever with any of his family, who are subject to the same restrictions as himself, unless upon medical subjects, and then only when sent for; and when finished, you are to leave them. You have no business to go amongst them, unless for medical purposes. Have you, Sir, had any communication with any of them unless upon those subjects?"

O'Meara answered by reminding the Governor of his own orders that, when visiting them, he should confine himself to medical matters.

"That reply, Sir, as usual, is not a direct one." He then moved on to say he did not approve of O'Meara's going into town when ships arrived: "You go to collect news for General Bonaparte." O'Meara simply said that he was a British officer and would not give up his rights. Anyway, he said, he wanted the opportunity, like everyone else, to buy the necessities of life as soon as they were landed and before there was a get-together to increase the price.

"If you intend to prohibit me from going to town, I must request orders to that effect in writing."

The Governor refused saying, with a sneer: "That request is worthy of the place you came from [Longwood], and the people with whom you associate. I do not think a person, under a pledge to Napoleon Bonaparte, should be received into company, and I certainly do not approve of your going into town when ships arrive. You are suspected by me, Sir."

"I am under no pledge to Napoleon, other than one which is tacitly understood in every gentleman's society."

"You are presumptuous and insolent to dare to judge of the line of conduct that His Majesty's Government has thought proper to pursue with regard to Napoleon Bonaparte."

"I do not attempt to judge of that, I merely mentioned what was the custom of society."

"You are a suspected man, Sir, you are suspected by *me*."

"I cannot help that, Sir. It is a consolation to me, however, under such circumstances, to have the moral high ground," which the Governor regarded as a fresh insult and rewarded O'Meara with another volley of abuse.

The final gubernatorial onslaught of the visit was poorly planned. "You took the opportunity, Sir, of staying in town the other day, when a ship arrived, instead of coming here to report, as you ought to have done."

"It was in compliance with your own instructions, Sir, of the thirtieth of January. You then told me, in the presence of Major Gorrequer, that when I saw Mr Baxter or Sir Thomas Reade in town, it might supersede the need for me to come to Plantation House on that day. Since I had already seen Mr Baxter that day and told him all there was to tell, I did not think it necessary to come up here."

While the Governor was trying to wriggle out of that one, O'Meara appealed to the ever-present Gorrequer if he had not repeated Lowe's words correctly. This was promptly construed as yet another insult and brought forth a fresh and prolonged paroxysm of invective.

Two months passed with the Governor quietly simmering away, trying to impose a doctor of his choice on Napoleon, and O'Meara keeping a low profile. All the while Napoleon's health continued its slow deterioration. London, however, continued to believe he was in good shape and that it was the French who were spreading rumours to the contrary.

Then, on April 4, the extent of the Governor's duplicity became apparent.

A resident foreigner on the island was chatting to Montholon and remarked on the Emperor's good health as reported in that day's bulletin. Montholon, knowing full well that O'Meara was no longer issuing bulletins, asked around and discovered that fraudulent bulletins were being prepared at the Governor's command by someone who can never have seen Napoleon. They were designed to show that the Governor was keeping a watchful eye on the General's health and that whatever else might be the matter with him, it could in no way be attributed to the Governor's negligence or to the climate of St Helena. Their most important recipients were the Commissioners. When, eventually, Bertrand demanded an explanation, the Governor told him that they merely repeated O'Meara's conversations with Baxter!

However, Sir Hudson Lowe's moment of triumphant inspiration came on April 10. Having failed in his application to London to have O'Meara removed from the island, he had Reade write to the doctor informing him that he was forbidden to leave Longwood. No reasons were given for this imposition of even more arbitrary restrictions than those imposed on the French. Since no one was allowed to enter Longwood without a pass, O'Meara was thus deprived of English society. In fact he was effectively deprived of society as a whole since the Governor had already prohibited him from all communications with the French, except on medical matters – and this he was able to enforce thanks to his ubiquitous spy network.

O'Meara was not the man to take this lying down. He immediately went to The Briars intending to lay the whole matter before Admiral Plampin who sent word by his secretary refusing to see him. Faced with this treatment from his commanding officer, O'Meara, in despair, was driven to write to the Governor tendering his resignation and to Bertrand explaining why he had been driven to take this ultimate step.

Napoleon sent for O'Meara on the fourteenth to grant him an audience prior to his anticipated departure. In French, he said:

"Well, doctor, so you are going to leave us. Will the world appreciate that it has been foolish enough to behave criminally towards my physician? Since you are now no more than a simple lieutenant subject to arbitrary power and military discipline, you no longer have the necessary independence for your services to be useful to me. I thank you for your care. Now leave this abode of shadows and sin. I shall die on that miserable bed, eaten up by disease and with no succour. And your country will be for ever dishonoured by my death."

The Governor yet again tried to impose another doctor on Napoleon, but Napoleon would have nothing to do with anyone associated with him. Eventually, the Commissioners made him understand that should Napoleon die while O'Meara, without being charged with anything, was in confinement or while Napoleon was under the care of a surgeon forced on him, people in Europe would begin to suspect that all was not as it seemed. Indeed, Balmain told him that the English would be accused of having poisoned the General and "millions of men will henceforth look upon you as his assassin." When the Commissioners emphasized that they themselves would be unable to give a satisfactory explanation, the Governor at last saw sense and released O'Meara. In his letter authorizing this, Lowe was obliged to acknowledge O'Meara as Napoleon's private surgeon, something, as I told you, he had previously contested.

These discussions with the Commissioners all took place at Plantation House, and on one occasion the Governor let rip at Baron Stürmer. The Baron calmly made him stop in front of a large mirror and begged him to contemplate his own features, adding that he could not wish to give his court a better representation of what was happening on St Helena than the figure in the mirror in front of him.

Before allowing O'Meara to resume his medical duties, Napoleon made him agree to write a report once a week, or more frequently if necessary, so as to put a stop to the production of any more fabricated bulletins. A copy of these reports was to be given to the Governor should he so wish. When O'Meara told Lowe about this arrangement, not only did he not wish it, but he forbade O'Meara giving him any written reports at all.

O'Meara's first report on being allowed to practise medicine again noted that the pain in the right side of his patient's abdomen was gradually getting worse, so much so that he actually asked O'Meara to resume his treatment: the obligatory exhortation to take exercise was so much wasted breath since Napoleon had not been out of his apartment for almost six weeks.

This confusing and thoroughly unsatisfactory situation was gathering impetus. The officers of the 53rd had elected O'Meara an honorary member of their mess, and that honour had been continued by the 66th. Towards the end of June, Lieutenant-Colonel Edmund Lascelles, their commanding officer, was visited, at the behest of the Governor, by Reade. He told the Colonel that since O'Meara had become "displeasing to the sight of the Governor", his officers should expel him from their mess as being unfit for their society. (Reade loved his job when he was required to deliver messages like this!) He further insinuated that such an action would be very agreeable to Sir Hudson, who would consider any person associating with O'Meara as his personal enemy.

Lascelles chose Lieutenant Rodolphus Reardon, a friend of O'Meara, to be the bearer of this sorry news and to beg him to resign of his own accord. But O'Meara was not prepared to be so obliging. He reckoned that if he did resign, his enemies would maintain he had done so because his conduct had compelled the members to throw him out. That evening, Lascelles came to see him but O'Meara wouldn't change his mind. Only by a vote of the mess or by order of the Governor would he renounce the honour.

When this reply was transmitted to Lowe, the next move was a foregone conclusion. Lowe sent an order by General Bingham to Lascelles instructing him to exclude O'Meara from the mess. Lascelles's letter to O'Meara was brief, to the point and gave no reason. An exchange of letters between O'Meara and the mess president expressed sorrow, respect, gratitude and friendship on both sides.

Lowe really was overstepping the mark with this insult to the 66th. Honorary membership of a mess had a deeper significance than is immediately apparent. But everyone from General Bingham downwards knew that if they didn't toe the line their time on St Helena was at an end and perhaps even their careers. Lascelles, as commanding officer of the regiment, was sent home but was allowed to return in 1820. Reardon was not so lucky; he was sent home for having talked to the Bertrands about O'Meara's dismissal, using the occasion to criticize the Governor's conduct; he was refused a return to the regiment and landed up joining the 49th Foot. The final exchange of letters summed up the true feelings of all concerned.

On July 9, seeing the way events were moving, O'Meara sat down and composed a comprehensive bulletin on Napoleon's health starting from September 1817. It told the story of a man who was far from well.

For a start he was still suffering with scurvy and was still troubled by swollen and painful legs. Infectious hepatitis (or at least something wrong with the liver) was supported by the presence of jaundice as indicated by the yellow whites of his eyes. More intriguing, though, was what appeared to be the presence of cholecystitis, to judge by a tender swelling in the upper right abdomen accompanied by pain in the right shoulder. There was nothing that would indicate with certainty anything seriously wrong with his stomach; dyspepsia could point to anything or nothing; we have to wait and see how things develop.

O'Meara's next report, and his last, came on July 25 and simply said he had visited Napoleon, whose malady was by no means altered for the better. Returning to his room, he was met by Captain Blakeney who gave him a letter from Colonel Wynyard, Lowe's military secretary:

"Sir, – I am directed by Lieutenant General Sir Hudson Lowe to inform you, that by an instruction received from Earl Bathurst, dated the 16th of May, 1818, he has been directed to withdraw you from your attendance upon General Buonaparte, and to *interdict you all further interviews with the inhabitants of Longwood.*

"Rear-Admiral Plampin has received instructions from the Lords Commissioners of the Admiralty as to your destination when you quit this island.

"You are in consequence to leave Longwood immediately after receiving this letter, without holding any further communication whatsoever with the persons residing there."

Lord Bathurst's hand in Plampin's instructions from the Lords Commissioners is all too apparent.

Once again O'Meara was having nothing to do with an order from the Governor. Regardless of the consequences, it was his professional duty towards a sick man to prescribe a regimen and to prepare the medicines that would be needed in the absence of a surgeon – which was likely to be quite lengthy since he was perfectly sure Napoleon still would accept no one who had anything to do with the Governor.

His duty completed, he went straight to Napoleon's apartment to tell him what had happened.

"Your minister is rash," was the response, "when the Pope was in France, I would sooner have cut off my right arm than have signed an order for the removal of his surgeon." He then gave him some commissions to fulfil when he reached Europe.

As a final gesture, he presented him with a superb snuff box and a statue of himself, shook his hand and embraced him saying: "*Adieu, O'Meara, nous ne nous reverrons encore. Soyez heureux.*"

However, any thought of happiness had to be delayed because when he got back to his room, Wynyard immediately escorted him from Longwood. His room was then searched in the vain hope that compromising documents might be found; his desk was forced and his trunks ransacked. Nothing incriminating was found although money and jewels, including a gold watch with chain and seals, an onyx ring, a diamond ring and other treasures, all presents from the Emperor and of great sentimental value, had disappeared. O'Meara protested to Admiral Plampin and a half-hearted investigation was carried out with Sir George Bingham as sitting magistrate. O'Meara was not allowed to see the report and the property was never recovered.

On July 26 Montholon wrote to the Governor:

"Yesterday Dr O'Meara left Longwood, forced to abandon his patient in the midst of the treatment which he was directing. This morning that treatment ceased; this morning a great crime began to be committed. The Emperor will never receive any physician other than Dr. O'Meara because he is his doctor."

He received a reply that same day:

"…. I shall not degrade myself or my nation by condescending to reply…. If Mr O'Meara's medical attendance was so desirable, he should have combined it with due respect and obedience to the orders and regulations of his Government in other points. The last act of his at Longwood was the breach of an order and the refusal to acknowledge the authority by which it was given.

"If Napoleon Buonaparte denies access to any other persons than Count Bertrand and yourself, reflect, Sir, on the responsibility which may thus attach to you. I am perfectly prepared to meet any which may fall to my share."

So swift had been O'Meara's expulsion from the island – he sailed on August 2 – that he was given no time to dispose of his property and settle with his creditors; he had to ask his fellow officers to do this for him. But when they presented the merchant with a bill drawn on his account, he refused to take it.

"In any country but this," he said, "I should be most happy to cash a bill on Mr O'Meara, but if the news of my having done so reaches the Governor's ears, he would certainly send me off the island." And Lowe's spies would certainly have ensured that it did reach his ears. The next day Stokoe presented the bill, this time drawn on his own account, and all was well – though in so doing he ensured that the enduring enmity of the Governor was drawn to himself.

On his return to England, O'Meara was dismissed the service, without pension.

* * *

On October 28, 1818, O'Meara wrote an official letter to the Lords of the Admiralty; here is an extract:

> "I think it my duty to state, as his late medical attendant, that considering the disease of the liver with which he is afflicted, the progress it has made in him, and reflecting on the great mortality produced by that complaint in the island of St. Helena, (so strongly exemplified in the number of deaths in the 66th regiment, the St. Helena Regiment, the squadron, and Europeans in general, and particularly in his majesty's ship Conqueror, which ship has lost about one sixth of her complement, nearly the whole of whom died within the last eight months,) it is my opinion, that the life of Napoleon Bonaparte will be endangered by a longer residence in such a climate as that of St. Helena, especially if that residence be aggravated by a continuance of those disturbances and irritations to which he has been hitherto subjected, and of which it is the nature of his distemper to render him particularly susceptible."

In 1821, when Napoleon was seriously ill, O'Meara wrote to Lord Bathurst offering to return to St Helena to give what help he could. The offer was rejected.

On the publication of his memoirs, *A Voice from St. Helena*, in 1822, O'Meara was sued for libel by Sir Hudson Lowe. The case dragged on until eventually the statute of limitations applied and the suit was dropped. However, O'Meara had to pay the costs on a technicality.

O'Meara died on June 10, 1836. Three days later, *The Courier* published a leading obituary which began:

> "The Island of St. Helena has given to Mr O'Meara a place in history, and when time shall have permitted all personal feeling to subside, history will do him justice. She will record him as a man of the most rigid integrity, capable of any sacrifice in the support of principle, and with a practical chivalry defying power, and welcoming privation in the maintenance of his proud consistency."

Barry Edward O'Meara was buried in the Parish Church of Paddington on June 18, 1836.

* * *

And now, *mon ami(e)*, you understand why the medical management of Napoleon Bonaparte fell apart at the seams so disastrously. The Emperor was not a well man and although O'Meara tried to do his best until he was shipped home, he was thwarted by the Governor and treated as piggy-in-the-middle in the bloody-minded contest between Lowe and Napoleon, to the extent that Napoleon refused to consult him and Lowe confined him to quarters for four weeks. It was a situation that could not continue and O'Meara was removed from the island by order of Lord Bathurst. His commanding officer, Admiral Plampin, behaved in an unforgivable manner and slammed the door in his face; he had other things on his mind than doing his duty of protecting the interests of a medical officer in the Royal Navy. And remember that none of this would have happened if he had not brought his mistress with him.

~17~
The realization of Stokoe's worst fears

(AUGUST, 1818 – JANUARY, 1819)

And now it's Stokoe's turn and he had already earned himself an unwelcome number of black marks from both Governor and Admiral. The Governor, in particular, was most evilly disposed towards him – remember Capri. And the Admiral was not prepared to forgive him for his insulting behaviour on board the *Northumberland*. Stokoe was dropped into this pernicious environment by his sense of duty as a doctor.

O'Meara's bed was not even cold before the Governor had installed James Verling in his room at Longwood. Verling was, you will recall, surgeon to the company of Royal Artillery stationed on St Helena, and had come out on a troopship in the convoy led by the *Northumberland*. He was another Irishman and had studied medicine at Dublin and Edinburgh, obtaining the Edinburgh MD at the early age of twenty-three. On joining the Army Ordnance Medical Department he soon found himself embroiled in the Peninsular War, from which he returned with five clasps to his Peninsular medal. He was thus a surgeon with the sort of military history that should have appealed to Napoleon. Regrettably, any appeal he might have had was well and truly annulled by his association with Sir Hudson Lowe. He was probably also the best and most competent doctor on the island.

Lowe had miscalculated badly in thinking he could replace O'Meara with Verling. In spite of living along the corridor for the next fourteen months Verling's only relationship with Napoleon was second-hand by virtue of his becoming medical attendant to the other French inhabitants of Longwood. Lowe was in despair. Whatever scheme he devised for getting Verling into Bonaparte's presence was thwarted, usually by Bertrand who protected his master like a mother lion her cubs.

When it finally dawned on him that Verling's chances of getting to see Napoleon, professionally or otherwise, were as remote as the Isles of the Blest, the Governor began to obsess again about someone actually seeing him every day. He discussed this problem with Montholon so often that in the middle of October Montholon came to Captain Nicholls's room and told him his children were playing under the Emperor's window and he might get a sight of him as he sometimes threw up the sash and spoke to them. He didn't. However, a day or two later Madame Montholon was in the garden with her children and this time Napoleon did open the window to chat to her. Nicholls, the most recent orderly officer at Longwood, watched him with his glass from behind the wall.

What he saw was a man with a greasy complexion wearing a dirty looking morning gown and a reddish handkerchief tied round his head. For some reason, best known to himself, Nicholls was left with the impression of having seen a ghost. Verling managed to catch a distant glimpse of him from the bottom of the Longwood garden, and even from that distance thought he looked very ill. After comparing notes with Nicholls he wrote to Baxter who sent a most intriguing reply:

"I am glad you had a sight of the man or ghost, but could have wished you were a little nearer. The time approaches when I think you will be in daily attendance on him, and it would not be surprising if I was also to be of the party….

"…. I like the proceedings of Montholon and it appears to be the wish of all parties to come to an understanding. I trust you entertain no doubt of B. selecting you as his immediate medical attendant; when he has once decided on that matter, my visits to you shall be more frequent as I shall then be quite free from every suspicion of a wish to obtrude my services…."

Little did Baxter understand the wishes of any party. The only party whose interests he did understand were those of Dr Alexander Baxter. Couldn't he get it into his thick head that 'B' would never select a medical attendant, no matter how good a doctor he might be, who had even the least connection with the Governor?

About a month later, in the middle of November, Stokoe must have thought that Christmas had come early that year. O joy! A French doctor was being sent out to replace O'Meara although it was not yet known when he would arrive. Ever since O'Meara's departure Stokoe had been living in mortal dread of attracting the Governor's unwelcome attention, particularly should he be called upon to attend Napoleon. He could now breathe a little more freely.

O, wretched man! Stokoe's worst fears were realized at daybreak on Sunday, January 17, 1819. He received the following note from Bertrand written at 1am:

"The Emperor has just had a sudden and violent attack. You are the only medical man at present in this country in whom he has shown any confidence. I beg you not to lose a moment in hastening to Longwood. On your arrival ask for me. I hope you will arrive in the course of the night. I am much troubled."

Even the summons did not arrive in the course of the night because Captain Nicholls had sent it by dragoon to the Governor at Plantation House who sent it on to the Admiral, a log asleep in the arms of his mistress at The Briars. He, in turn, sent it to the officer on duty in the harbour who had to take a boat out to the *Conqueror* where the captain's secretary took the time to write a covering note for Captain Stanfell (who had succeeded John Davie as captain of the *Conqueror*):

"The Admiral has desired me to say that you are to order Mr. Stokoe to go directly to Longwood and call on Dr. Verling, as

Buonaparte is very ill."

A ribbon of bloody red tape. Cut it at your peril!

But even the Governor had not been the first to see what should have been treated as both urgent and confidential. Nicholls had first woken Verling at about 3am to show him Bertrand's letter.

When Stokoe did eventually receive the summons, he knew he had no alternative but to get to Longwood with all possible speed. There was just no way he could duck the obligation. He was well and truly ensnared in the web woven by two venomous spiders.

He arrived at Longwood at 6.45am and called on Verling to ask him to be in readiness should he be needed. He then crossed to the Bertrand's villa to report to the Grand Marshal. The attack, he was told, began with a sharp pain in the right side of the abdomen and in the shoulders, accompanied by a violent fever, and followed by oppression and giddiness. He was unconscious for a few minutes. It was at this moment that Bertrand had written his letter.

The attack had, however, been relieved by a hot bath and Napoleon was out of immediate danger. He was now sleeping and Stokoe was asked to wait and see him when he awoke. The Bertrands gave him breakfast and afterwards Montholon joined them to propose that he should replace O'Meara and become the Emperor's surgeon. Stokoe declined – are you surprised?

He was asked why. In answer he said that it was an appointment he would have unhesitatingly accepted had he not seen the way O'Meara had been persecuted which, O'Meara had told him, was because he had refused to degrade himself by becoming a spy for the Governor. Montholon promptly disappeared from the room. He returned in about an hour with a paper containing eight Articles, no doubt dictated by Napoleon.

These eight Articles effectively covered all the difficulties that had so aggrieved O'Meara. They dealt with what would be Stokoe's position and authority, and how he would be protected from the Governor's actions. He would write two copies of a daily, or more frequent, bulletin on Napoleon's health; one for Longwood, the other for the Governor should he require it – this was to a put a stop to the false bulletins that someone, probably Baxter, was still preparing. Restrictions on his written and verbal communications with the French would be lifted and he would not be compelled to report to the Governor anything he saw or heard at Longwood, unless it might compromise his oath of allegiance.

They concluded with: "In accepting these conditions, Mr Stokoe is to preserve the integrity of all his rights as an English citizen and officer. He demands to receive from the Admiralty the same pay as his predecessor, and not to be assimilated in any way with the French prisoners. The whole of the above to be done with the permission of his chief, Rear-Admiral Plampin."

Stokoe saw nothing in the Articles incompatible with his honour and told Montholon that he would accept the appointment if both the Admiral and the Governor consented to the conditions.

At length he was taken in to see Napoleon who was lying on a sofa. His skin was sallow and his features drawn. The pain in his side was still there and the slightest pressure over the spot made him cry out. At the end of a careful examination, Stokoe diagnosed a chronic condition of the liver.

"How long might a man live with such a complaint?" Napoleon asked.

"There are instances of men living to an advanced age."

"Yes, but is one likely to live to that age in a tropical climate?"

"No," was the blunt answer.

The Emperor clenched his fist and shouted, with passion, "I should have lived to the age of eighty if they had not brought me to this vile place."

In his official bulletin on the visit, Stokoe wrote:

"I found the patient in a very weak state, complaining of considerable pain in the right side, in the region of the liver, and with shooting pain in the right shoulder. About midnight he had been suddenly seized with violent pains in the head, succeeded by vertigo and syncope, which continued nearly a quarter of an hour. After recovering from this state, he had recourse to a warm bath, which produced violent perspiration and relieved him immediately.

"From the evident determination of blood to the head, it will be highly necessary that a medical man should be near his person, in order that immediate assistance may be afforded in case of a recurrence of the above alarming symptoms, as well as for the daily treatment of chronic hepatitis, which the above symptoms indicate."

[Between you and me, these symptoms more probably indicate an attack of cholecystitis and the passage of a gallstone down the biliary duct into his duodenum and from thence into the wide world outside. At this date disease of the gallbladder was not recognized as such and was lumped together with disease of the liver, but the pain that made Napoleon cry out when Stokoe pressed over a certain spot certainly suggests that he was pressing over an inflamed gallbladder. The pain in the shoulder was probably referred from the gallbladder. I am reluctant, however, to speculate on the nature of "the determination of blood to the head". As it doesn't fit with my concept of a cerebrovascular accident, I like to think of it as a component of this attack of biliary colic, particularly as it never recurred.]

Stokoe eventually managed to get away from Longwood at two o'clock. On his way back to his ship he called at The Briars and handed the Admiral the document containing the Articles. Plampin saw nothing to object to – but would not give a definite decision until he had talked it over with the Governor. However, events were ahead of him. Bertrand had already given Captain Nicholls a copy of the Articles to forward to the Governor, adding that Napoleon was willing to take Dr Stokoe as his physician on these terms and that Dr Stokoe had consented to attend on Napoleon provided both Governor and Admiral agreed.

Lowe, bloody-minded as ever, took umbrage. He had not heard from Stokoe since he had left for Longwood; indeed, had he even got there and seen General Bonaparte? What arguments had the French used to persuade him to agree to such proposals? These Articles were not the sort of thing that sprang out of the thin air of a sudden call at a late hour – and without any prior reference to the Admiral or himself. He then put all these considerations in writing and sent them to Plampin.

Lowe evidently suspected that some mysterious plot was being hatched at Longwood in which Stokoe was implicated. After all, he had failed to call on him on his way back from Longwood and, moreover, he had acted with suspicious haste. Although Nicholls had told him of Stokoe's reservations, it suited Lowe better to regard a conditional arrangement as a done deal.

That evening Napoleon's staff were hopping around like scalded cats in their anxiety over Napoleon's condition. Stokoe had said that it was "highly desirable" for a medical man to be close to him – and the only acceptable doctor was Stokoe himself. So, in pitch darkness and pouring rain, Montholon and Nicholls set off for Plantation House, escorted by two men carrying lanterns. In the library at ten o'clock, Montholon put it to the Governor that until he had come to a decision over Stokoe and the Articles, he should allow him to stay at Longwood. Stokoe was then called in.

Not taking his eyes off the doctor, Montholon went on to say he was convinced the Emperor would have another 'apoplectic' attack that night and it was essential to have a surgeon at hand to bleed him. And it was no use the Governor arguing that Verling already was on hand as he well knew that Mr Stokoe was the only medical man in whom the Emperor had confidence.

Lowe gave the impression that he was not averse to this arrangement but explained that Stokoe was under the Admiral's authority and that he (Lowe) could not dispose of his services. The misbegotten hypocrite! To deny the powers he possessed now that the Admiral was screwed down under his thumb, and to reprimand Stokoe for not having reported to him when he had already reported to the Admiral "under whose authority" he was, was quite beyond the pale. But he was not yet done.

Montholon argued that the Governor represented the Prince Regent on the island and so could give orders to anybody. Lowe countered with the observation that the naval commander-in-chief, the head of another service, was entirely independent of him and he (the Governor) could give no orders to persons under his (the Admiral's) authority. He would, however, confer with the Admiral. In the meantime Mr Stokoe would, he said, be at Longwood the next morning. Plantation House stubbornly refused to believe in the seriousness of Napoleon's illness – only with his dying breath would they admit that he really was ill. The meeting closed without result and the Emperor without a doctor for the night.

Napoleon, however, had another violent attack of pain before Montholon returned and Bertrand had no alternative but to send an urgent message to the Governor demanding Stokoe's presence. Mercifully, Stokoe had used his initiative and had been with his patient since 6am. Mercifully, because the Governor had chosen to hold the letter for twelve hours until midday on Monday, the eighteenth; he had made up his mind to take no further notice of "those people at Longwood".

Lowe was sailing too close to the wind for his own good over this matter of Napoleon's doctor. Four months previously he had received a letter from Lord Bathurst giving him orders that O'Meara should be replaced by any surgeon on the island approved of by Napoleon. Stokoe was that surgeon. Yet Lowe chose to ignore the order despite the risk of incurring Bathurst's wrath should he find out. He still believed he would be able to get a replacement into Longwood who would report to him every word spoken by Napoleon, every detail of events in Longwood – in effect to be his spy in the General's camp. And Stokoe was the last man who would undertake such a despicable role.

Stokoe's second examination of Napoleon confirmed his findings of the day before. In his second bulletin he reported:

"It appears from the symptoms of chronic hepatitis (the first appearance of which he experienced sixteen months ago) that this is the principal cause of the present derangement in his health, and although they are described as having increased considerably of late, yet, judging from present appearances, I do not apprehend any immediate danger, although it must be presumed that in a climate where the above disease is so prevalent it will eventually shorten his life.

"The more alarming symptom is that which was experienced on the night of the 16th, a recurrence of which may soon prove fatal, particularly if medical assistance is not at hand."

On his way back Stokoe, as before, reported to The Briars. There was a distinct frost in the atmosphere. When he was shown into the office, the Admiral was seated behind his desk as expected but, in the middle of the room, sitting doing nothing, was his secretary. So unusual was this that Stokoe instantly realized the man was there as a witness. The Admiral proceeded to ask about everything that had happened and everything that had been said at Longwood. With that out of the way he went on to enquire about Napoleon's health and to make notes while Stokoe recited his report from memory – he had left the actual document at Longwood.

The interview over, Stokoe was ordered not to visit Longwood again without a pass.

That Monday evening Gorrequer wrote to Nicholls telling him that the Governor and the Admiral had had a pow wow. Plampin had made the point that if Stokoe were to attend at Longwood, he should not be entirely removed from the (naval) squadron. For his part, the Governor had no objection to Stokoe continuing to attend Napoleon Bonaparte whenever required, but he wanted the visits to be made in company with Verling.

Stokoe was summoned for the third time by Bertrand on the

afternoon of Tuesday, January 19. As ordered, he called on Plampin for a pass. The Admiral had just returned from a session with the Governor and was primed with fresh instructions. So, despite Stokoe's being on his way to see a desperately ill man, he was subjected to a repeat catechism of the previous day but considerably more searching, and again with the Admiral's secretary recording the proceedings . When Plampin had run out of questions regarding the Articles, he turned to the bulletin and Napoleon's health, treating Stokoe like a final-year student, and confidently disputing with him the facts of the illness. First he challenged the medical history Stokoe had taken. He then queried whether he had actually seen and felt what he had described, and then challenged the reliability of his conclusions. Finally Stokoe was chastised for having omitted General Bonaparte's name from the bulletins. This was, Stokoe said, because when he asked Bertrand what he should put, he was told 'Napoleon' or 'the patient'. However, as he knew the Governor demanded 'General Buonaparte', he felt that to put no name at all was the most diplomatic solution. The Admiral didn't agree.

Stokoe eventually got his pass and reached Longwood at about 6pm. Nicholls showed him Gorrequer's letter asking that Verling should be present, but everyone knew it was useless to try. Stokoe was now well and truly caught between Scylla and Charybdis. If he disobeyed orders and obeyed his conscience he was playing into the Governor's hands; if he obeyed orders by refusing to visit Napoleon alone and fatal complications set in after he had left Longwood, the Governor would hold him to blame – "A wish, Mr Stokoe, is not a command." He could hear the words being spoken.

Bertrand's anxiety for his master had by no means been exaggerated. Stokoe found him much deteriorated. His pulse rate indicated that there had been a remarkably rapid rise in the fever, and the character of the hepatitis seemed to be changing, probably, Stokoe thought, because a chronic condition had become acute.

Fearing that "the violent tendency of the blood to the head" heralded a return of Sunday night's attack, he decided to spend the night at Longwood.

To forestall the anticipated attack, Stokoe begged the patient to allow himself to be bled, but Napoleon waved the idea aside. Towards 5am, however, with his headache almost unbearable, the Emperor consented. The relief was slight.

Stokoe would gladly have spent the whole of Wednesday, January 20, at Longwood, but at midday he was summoned back to The Briars where he handed the Admiral his report, which ended with:

"I took this opportunity of more particularly examining the liver, and am fully persuaded of the diseased state of that viscus, having distinctly felt a degree of hardness.... I therefore advised the immediate adoption of a course of mercury, with other medicines in such form as best suited the constitution of the patient."

But Stokoe had reached the end of his tether. When he got back to his ship he immediately wrote to the Admiral:

"The experience of today points to the necessity of my declining all further communication with Longwood.

"I therefore humbly beg leave that, in case my services are again demanded in aid of General Bonaparte, you will be pleased to cause Count Bertrand to be acquainted with my wishes on this head."

No sooner was the letter written than Stokoe received yet another call to Longwood. To try to settle the matter there and then, he delivered the letter himself to The Briars. Regrettably, the Admiral was at dinner and wouldn't see him. He merely sent a message ordering Stokoe to go to Longwood and spend the night there. He did, however, instruct him to return the next day without fail and by the latest at half-past-ten. In making these instructions so precise was the Admiral deliberately seeking to entrap Stokoe by ensuring he would be late and consequently would be disobeying orders? If that indeed was his intention, he succeeded.

Stokoe rode through the gates of The Briars at midday on the Wednesday, two hours late. It was not his fault. The Emperor had asked him to extend the consultation, and then on his way back he had fallen from his horse, so bad were the tracks after the recent rainstorms.

He immediately reported to Admiral Plampin (the Admiral's secretary present): "I saw General Bonaparte yesterday," he began, "and his fever was slight, but he complained that the pain in his side was worse. This morning the pain was still there and almost as bad.

"I recommended a warm bath, which he took immediately, and was still in it when I left.

"I told him that he should immediately start a course of medicines, some of which I had already prepared and would send others from town, with instructions, as I could no longer continue my visits to Longwood under the circumstances I was subjected to. I also told him that I had already asked you to make known my wishes on that head to Count Bertrand. He replied that he would take no medicine that he did not receive from the hands of his own surgeon."

He went on to leave the Admiral in no doubt that he was finished with the malignant situation he had been manoeuvred into. Did they want him to continue as General Bonaparte's medical attendant, or did they not?

By way of reply, Admiral Plampin assumed the mantle of Sir Hudson:

"What kept you so long after the time I told you to be back here?"

"General Bonaparte wished me to stay."

"So you disobeyed my order because General Bonaparte wished you to remain at Longwood!"

"He wanted me to stay so that I could see the effect of the

warm bath."

"Was General Bonaparte so ill that you found your presence absolutely necessary?"

"No I cannot say he was that ill, but he wanted me to stay."

"Then because General Bonaparte wanted you to stay, you disobeyed my command. I ordered you to be here at half-past ten this morning. It appears you consider General Bonaparte's wishes overrule any order of mine."

"Would you have had me leave him?"

"Certainly, as you do not think your presence was absolutely necessary. You ought to have obeyed my order; neither necessity nor humanity required your staying."

The second misbegotten hypocrite on the island was as good at the job as his teacher. The agreement between Governor and Admiral was something that needed to be kept on a need-to-know basis – and no-one needed to know! Nevertheless, the admirable Gorrequer would have known (or guessed), but he knew how to keep his mouth shut; Reade would almost certainly have known otherwise he could not have done his job properly as deputy adjutant general on the island. For the rest…? But the two naval surgeons most concerned had not the faintest idea.

Not being one to leave unanswered correspondence lying around, the Admiral chose that evening to answer the letter Stokoe had delivered to him the previous day when he was at dinner:

"….I have only to observe that it's of no consequence for me to know what experience you yesterday gained, nor do I consider it requisite for you to ask my leave to decline your services in aid of General Bonaparte, which I have never yet commanded. And, never having had any correspondence with Count Bertrand, I cannot condescend to commence one with him for the mere purpose of conveying your wishes on that head…."

So hypocritical and divorced from reality was this convoluted text that Stokoe sought out Captain Stanfell to reassure himself of his sanity.

"Would you be good enough," he asked, "to grant me a second reading of the order sent you by the commander-in-chief on the morning of the seventeenth (Sunday) and delivered to me by you? It would seem, to judge from a letter I have just received from the Admiral, that in attending General Bonaparte I have misconceived my duty." The captain was too wily an old bird to be caught giving an answer to that one!

Dr Stokoe never again visited Longwood.

Balmain reported the situation to the Tsar: "He is the second English doctor dismissed from Longwood. With the exception of Baxter, who the French say is a poisoner; Verling, whom they will not see, and Livingstone, who is an accoucheur, there is none other to give them."

Lowe was, however, sufficiently disturbed by Stokoe's bulletins to show them to Baxter and ask for his comments. Baxter leapt at the opportunity for demonstrating his loyalty to the Governor. Indeed, so close to him was he that he sometimes addressed him as "Dear General" rather than the official "Sir" used by everyone else. Moreover, he was already hard at work discrediting the ill-informed belief that Napoleon really was ill.

Stokoe's bulletins were grist to his mill.

> "Dear General," (he began his written report.) "On Mr Stokoe's first visit he says he could neither see nor feel the swelling as Mr O'Meara had described it. He said the greatest danger was from apoplexy which could carry him off if medical aid was not available. In spite of this Stokoe recommended a more nourishing diet, which usually means animal food and wine. But such a diet ordered for a patient considered to be in danger of determination of blood to the head (apoplexy), makes one suspicious either of the sincerity or the professional talents of Mr Stokoe. On January 20 Mr Stokoe says he is fully convinced the liver is diseased, having felt a hardness. Mr O'Meara mentioned that there was an evident enlargement over the

region of the liver, but could not discover whether the liver was diseased on account of the extreme obesity.

"So Mr Stokoe cannot perceive the swelling and Mr O'Meara is unable to feel the hardness. Mr Stokoe on his first visit could neither find the hardness or the swelling, although the complaint had been on the increase for sixteen months."

There was nothing strictly inaccurate in his report, but Baxter certainly knew how to tweak the excerpts from the relevant bulletins to make it seem that the two doctors were unable to agree. Lowe was highly satisfied as the result added considerable weight to his official view that Napoleon was exaggerating his illness. The obscurity surrounding disease of the gall-bladder and gallstones didn't help matters either.

* * *

And now, *mon ami(e)*, you appreciate the appalling mess that was now Napoleon's medical management. However, it needn't have been had Lowe accepted Napoleon's choice of Stokoe to be his doctor, which in fact he had been told to do by Lord Bathurst. But no, he was prepared to face the wrath of London in the hope of getting his own man into Longwood. Stokoe was not to see the Emperor again.

~18~
The Royal Navy has no further interest in Longwood

(JANUARY – SEPTEMBER, 1819)

A few days after Stokoe's disagreement with Plampin, Captain Stanfell informed him that the Admiral intended to have him court-martialled. Astounded, Stokoe asked to know the charges.

"Contempt and disobedience of orders."

"Then I must hold the Admiral responsible for whatever I am charged with. His positive orders left me with no discretionary powers."

Stokoe now saw the Admiral's instructions for what they really were; they had left him little hope of escape without being guilty of disobeying orders. This, he now knew, was sheer vindictiveness on the Admiral's part because he refused to conform blindly to the Governor's wishes. Even so, he thought he might be able to avoid a court-martial.

He went to see Captain Stanfell again and told him he had been unable to attend to his naval duties for several days owing to the fall from his horse and, moreover, his health had suffered considerably from the climate. In view of this he asked the captain to tell the Admiral that he would willingly be invalided and quit the station.

The Admiral failed to respond and after two or three days Stanfell suggested Stokoe should apply for a medical board. This was granted and the next day he was ordered on board HMS *Trincomalee* bound for England. As he himself expressed it: "I thought all my sufferings at an end." Experience had taught him nothing.

Stokoe landed at Portsmouth on April 14 and found he had to submit to a second medical board at the Admiralty in London to confirm his sick leave. The examining physician was a Dr Weir, assisted by two other members of the board, one of whom was Sir George Cockburn. Dr Weir was an obvious plant. He made light of every complaint Stokoe produced and when he had finished wrote out his report and handed it to Sir George.

"This will do," said Sir George. Then turning to Stokoe, "Mr Stokoe, you may retire. I think it likely we shall send you back again."

On his way downstairs he met Sir Pulteney Malcolm. He told him he suspected he would be going back to St Helena but didn't relish the prospect of serving under Admiral Plampin again.

"Stokoe, you are a surgeon. You are more independent than any of us so long as you do your duty, but I think you ought to view your being sent back again as proof that your conduct has been approved of." This remark showed all too clearly that Sir Pulteney was ignorant of events on St Helena after he had handed over command to Sir Robert Pamplin – certainly of the Governor/Admiral agreement. At all events the unfortunate Stokoe was doomed. He was persona very much non grata with both the Government, through Lowe, and the Royal Navy, through Plampin. The members of the board had received their instructions. Stokoe was not to escape unpunished.

Little did John Stokoe, with only a few months to go to complete a service of twenty-five years, twenty as surgeon, and retire on ten shillings a day, appreciate that the political pond in which he was floundering was wider and deeper than any he could have imagined in his wildest dreams.

He was returned to St Helena on the *Abundance*, a storeship, which left Portsmouth on April 19 and arrived at Jamestown on August 21. He transferred to the *Conqueror* where his name was once again entered on the ship's books as surgeon. This was necessary to allow the important business of the day to proceed.

This began when the officer of the watch received a letter from Captain Stanfell – who was ashore in the admiral's office – directing him to put memorandum No. 22 into Stokoe's hands on the quarter deck. It contained the notification from the Admiralty that he was to be court-martialled. This was the sole reason he had been returned to St Helena. Virtually everything in speech, writing or action that Stokoe had had to do with Napoleon and the inhabitants of Longwood, and the records of his meetings with Admiral Plampin, was turned into one of the ten charges brought against him.

The court-martial met on August 30, on board the *Conqueror*.

Unaware of what was awaiting him and having been hustled on board the *Abundance* at Portsmouth, Stokoe had left all his relevant papers, letters and other documents behind in England. Moreover, he had to defend himself as no fellow officer was willing to act as his counsel – to do so would have compromised himself with the Governor. And he was not allowed to enforce the attendance of his two key witnesses, Bertrand and Montholon. Only two officers testified willingly: Lieutenant James Hay, to whom Stokoe had complained of falling from his horse; and William Clark, an assistant surgeon on board the *Conqueror*, who testified to finding a severe contusion on the shoulder as a result of the accident.

But perhaps the greatest stumbling-block Stokoe had to overcome was the British conviction that General Bonaparte was not really a sick man.

At the end of four days Stokoe was horrified to hear himself found guilty and to be dismissed the service. The spectres of Governor and Admiral hung miserably over the *Conqueror* that day. It might, though, have done his soul good had he learnt that during this short stay, Napoleon dictated three letters summoning "s*on chirurgien Stokoe*" to his side. Bertrand had slipped the letters into Nicholls's hand but for whatever reason they never reached the intended recipient.

Stokoe was sent back to England immediately after his conviction but, in consideration of his long service, his judges recommended the Admiralty to grant him half-pay (they believed he had been harshly and unfairly treated). However, as he was not exactly a retired officer, it was thought more appropriate that he should have a pension of three hundred pounds a year from the Civil List. Other pensions found their way to him, including one from the Bonapartes. Joseph, Napoleon's eldest brother, was a particular benefactor and the two men became personal friends.

Stokoe married late in life and his last years were saddened by the death, not only of his wife, but also of his two children, a son and a daughter. He died suddenly from a stroke on September 13, 1852.

* * *

And what of Admiral Plampin and his mistress? The Admiral's tour of duty ended ten months later in July, 1820, when he was relieved by Rear-Admiral Robert Lambert. In 1825 he was promoted Vice-Admiral and given command of the Irish Naval Station based at Cork. Not a bad reward for his truly reprehensible conduct on St Helena. He died in 1834 at the age of seventy-two and was buried at Wantage. Of his mistress all was silence until one day in the spring of 2010 she stepped out from historical darkness:

The marriage took place in the church of St George the Martyr, Southwark,on February 6, 1821, between Robert Plampin, bachelor, and Fanny Mitchell, spinster, both of this parish.

Fanny was twenty years younger than Sir Robert. She died in 1864 aged eighty-two and was also buried at Wantage; there were no children.

* * *

And so *mon ami(e)*, with Stokoe's departure from the island, the navy had no further interest in Longwood. But before we completely finish with Sir Robert Plampin, I must be sure you realize that you are among the very first to learn the identity of his mistress. Nevertheless, a certain air of mystery still surrounds her.

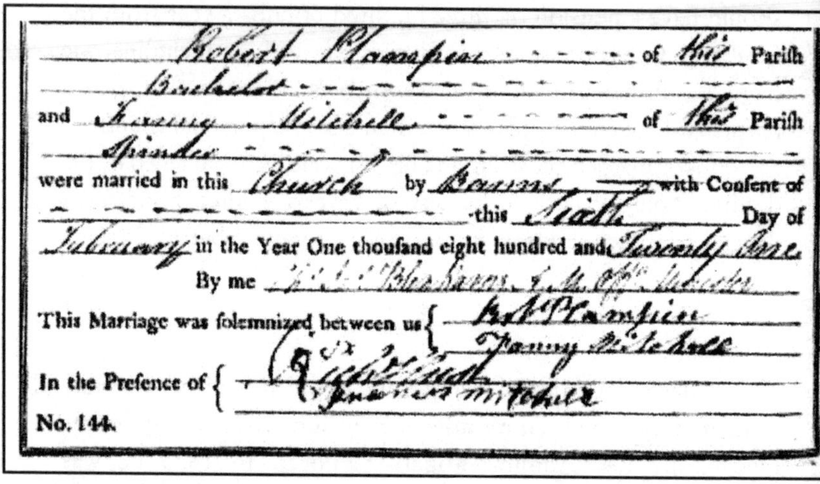

Robert Plampin of this Parish
Bachelor
and Fanny Mitchell of this Parish
Spinster
were married in this Church by Banns with Consent of
this Sixth Day of
February in the Year One thousand eight hundred and Twenty One
By me [illegible]
This Marriage was solemnized between us { Robt Plampin / Fanny Mitchell
In the Presence of { [illegible] / Frances Mitchell
No. 144.

Why didn't they marry before leaving for St Helena, or ask the Rev Boys to marry them (assuming he would have been willing to do so)? Why did Plampin take her with him to St Helena and live there openly together, when he would have been aware of the scandal this would cause? He was indeed fortunate that Lowe did not send them both packing back to England – though two decent naval surgeons could have wished that fortune had shone elsewhere. Or, the cynic might ask, was she, at the age of thirty-eight, worried that if she didn't go with him as his mistress, despite the humiliation, she might lose all hope of marriage? At any rate, on their return he did at least make an honest woman of her just as soon as he could.

~19~
The trials and tribulations of Francesco Antommarchi

(JANUARY – SEPTEMBER, 1819)

And now, *mon ami(e)*, having got the answer to our first question all safely tucked away, we can continue our search for the answers to the second – what actually killed the Emperor? And what else might he have been suffering from at the time?

* * *

Napoleon had been without a resident doctor for fourteen months. His only contact with the medical profession had been Stokoe's four visits six months previously which established that he really was a sick man (though this was not accepted by the English who believed it only when they saw him on his death-bed). During those six months his health had fluctuated with periods of reasonable well-being interspersed with episodes of abdominal pain and discomfort attributable primarily to the liver and gallbladder. Whether or not he took any of the medicines recommended by Stokoe must remain a moot point, though on past experience I fancy not. All-in-all he looked distinctly unhealthy.

Coming to his aid, as foretold more than a year ago – the heavy hand of bureaucracy rests on us all! – was the 'French' doctor aboard the ship that sailed into the Jamestown roads on the morning of September 18, 1819. The *Snipe*, an inferior trading brig with a cargo of flour and timber, was in very poor shape. She leaked and listed to port – but she had done that since leaving Gravesend the best part of two months before. Food and water were in seriously short supply since her captain had failed to lay in provisions at his last port of call where he had tried to sell his timber but without any luck. This made him so mad that the last thing he was going to do was waste money on his passengers' "inordinate appetites".

Besides the doctor the *Snipe* was carrying four other passengers and a motley lot they were, too. However, the prime object of the expedition was to provide Napoleon with a doctor he would trust, though I sense that Cardinal Fesch had different priorities.

From the word go, Dr Francesco Antommarchi has laboured under a poor reputation. Originally, this arose because he was an ardent Bonapartist at a time when Bonapartists were decidedly out of favour. Then, as history began to intrude, things went from bad to worse; in particular, he was accused of lack of clinical experience, and of being qualified only to perform Napoleon's post-mortem.

Born in Corsica in 1789, Antommarchi's curriculum vitae was, in fact, impeccable: he had trained at Pisa and Florence and in 1808 was awarded doctorates in philosophy and medicine by the University of Pisa; in 1812 he obtained a diploma in surgery. In 1818 he was demonstrator in anatomy at the University of Pisa under the renowned Professor Mascagni before being seconded to the hospital of Sainte-Marie Neuve in Florence. On his travel permit for St Helena he is described as having dark hair and eyes and being five feet, ten inches tall.

Among his acquaintances was Simeon Colonna who happened to be chamberlain to Madame Mère (Napoleon's mother) and, one day when discussing his future, Colonna suggested he could do worse than offer to go to St Helena. Confident his offer would be accepted, Antommarchi began settling his private affairs and ensuring that the anatomical atlas of his now late professor, Paolo Mascagni, would proceed unhindered to publication. Because of his well-known Bonapartist leanings, this behaviour led to his being suspected of subversive dealings: he was said to be Napoleon's agent, a danger to all Italy. The police became interested in what he was up to and he was threatened, informed against and generally persecuted. He asked for leave of absence from the University – it was refused. He tendered his resignation – it was not accepted. The more he argued, the greater the suspicion. The mere name of Napoleon filled people's minds with terror: nothing could dissipate their fears.

Getting nowhere, he appealed directly to Cardinal Joseph Fesch, Madame Mère's half-brother who looked after her affairs. He didn't have long to wait for an answer:

"I have been asked by Lord Bathurst," wrote Fesch from Rome on December 19, 1818, "to send a reputable surgeon to St Helena to attend the Emperor Napoleon. In view of your excellent testimonials and of the assurances I have received of your wish to serve him, I have selected you. You will, therefore, deliver the enclosed letter to Lord Burghersh, the British Minister in Florence, to obtain from him the necessary passports for travel to Rome and on through Germany to London.

"The sum required for the journey will be given you here [Rome] and the Emperor himself will fix your annual salary."

Antommarchi duly delivered the letter to Lord Burghesh; nevertheless, his persecution continued and he was very nearly arrested, but eventually he got his passports and arrived in Rome on January 7, 1819.

He was introduced to Madame Mère, the Cardinal and all the members of the imperial family then in Rome. His expectations of an early departure were dashed by the Cardinal who was beset by a multitude of doubts and scruples over the nomination of a priest to go with Antommarchi. He had been persuaded by persons of influence within the church to drop his first and most suitable choice. Still, the Lord would provide. Divine inspiration brought the Cardinal to his knees: a missionary would be the perfect choice

– St Helena was a Protestant island, ripe for conversion. He need look no further. Abbé Buonavita had been twenty-five years in Mexico and on his return to Europe had been almoner to Madame Mère on Elba and then chaplain to Princess Pauline, Napoleon's favourite sister, in Rome.

The Abbé had no hesitation about accepting the job. He was sixty-six and his travel permit gave his height as five feet, ten inches. So far so good. But read on and you will find a man who was feeble, gouty and infirm and had recently suffered a stroke that had left him almost entirely deprived of speech. We must now suspect that the Cardinal's primary concern was, indeed, the gathering of souls on St Helena (Buonavita had had an impressive record in Mexico); after that came Napoleon's spiritual well-being; his bodily health was none of the Cardinal's business.

The Cardinal had, however, overlooked the fact that missionaries were forbidden by the College of the Propaganda (*Congregation de propaganda fide)* to travel alone on missions that crossed the equator. Without wasting time, he chose Abbé Vignale to join the party. He was a man of about twenty-five and, by all accounts, low-born, ignorant and illiterate, though he had apparently studied medicine for three or four years. To complete the party Pauline gave her cook, Jacques Chandelier, a highly competent chef, described in his travel permit as thirty-one and five feet, three inches tall; and Madame Mère donated one of her manservants, Jacques Coursot described as thirty-four and five feet, ten inches tall.

Antommarchi had been in Rome nearly a month and his patience was wearing thin; he repeatedly asked, pleaded with, beseeched the Cardinal to fix the date of departure, but he wouldn't listen to reason. He was too deeply enmeshed in church affairs to worry about the expedition until the Abbé was fit to make the journey. The doctor would just have to curb his impatience. During the wait, however, O'Meara's last bulletin summarizing Napoleon's medical history on the island reached the imperial family. The Cardinal and Madame Mère together asked that it should be put before a meeting of some of the leading lights of Roman medicine who, after thorough discussion, produced a document which was to be Antommarchi's ultimate medical authority. It began by giving their opinion of the diagnosis: "The disease of the august patient consists in an obstruction of the liver and a tendency to scurvy."

It went on to describe the treatment to be given, beginning with general measures: "To treat the first mentioned, the diet should contain fresh vegetables, bitter or slightly acidic fruits, and easily digestible animal products designed to produce chyle [a fatty fluid formed in the intestine during digestion] of an emollient nature. Exercise in the open air, on foot, horseback or in a carriage; live in an airy situation, exposed to dry and healthy winds; and in general the use of mild remedies that do not irritate the system." Then came a list of the medicines that could, with advantage, be given depending on the presenting symptoms, and concluding with the advice that, in the hottest time of the year, cold or slightly tepid baths might be taken as well as shower-baths directed at the right hypochondrium. However, the shower-baths should be given with caution if the obstruction in the liver should increase, or the scurvy forbid its use. The document was dated 1 February, 1819. All in all a first class assessment by doctors who had not seen the patient – although the recommendations on exercise might meet with raised eyebrows from him and we all have a pretty good idea how the advice on where he should live would be received! The document also reflects the excellence of O'Meara's doctoring.

And still there were no signs of departure. Church matters continued to give the Cardinal other things to think about. When he did decide that Buonavita was fit enough to travel, two more days were lost while the imperial family threw a lavish farewell dinner party. The expedition, which resembled nothing so much as the cast of a Donizetti comic opera, departed on February 25. Their horses were bad; the roads were worse. They travelled slowly out of consideration for Abbé Buonavita. Eventually they arrived in London on April 19.

When they had gathered themselves they called on Lord Bathurst to deliver a letter from Cardinal Fesch explaining their mission, but he refused to see them and sent his secretary instead. A day or two later a letter arrived telling them to hold themselves in readiness to set off – but Vignali would not to be one of their number as Fesch had been given permission for a party of only four people. Buonavita therefore played the age and infirmity hand and persuaded his lordship to change his mind.

But the Fates, or someone acting on their behalf, conspired to stop them leaving; first, the winds were contrary, then there were no available sailings for St Helena. They would be sent out on the first transport available. However, Antommarchi knew that places could frequently be found – but it would never do for him to be seen as better informed than the Government, particularly as he was well aware that the delays were due to the British belief that the real object of the expedition was to study the possibilities of Napoleon's escape. Antommarchi's reputation had preceded him.

Quite by chance, O'Meara happened to be in London and Antommarchi wasted no time in visiting him. O'Meara confirmed that hepatitis was endemic on the island and that the Emperor was getting steadily worse; he regarded cure as impossible unless Napoleon were to be removed from the baleful influence of the climate. O'Meara regaled him with the full story of Stokoe's misfortunes and gave him copies of his various bulletins.

Antommarchi was spurred into action. Without asking for the secretary he went straight to Lord Bathurst's office. Reminding him of his promises, he told him he knew ships were ready to sail; these delays had to stop as the mission's expenses were mounting and the Emperor's condition deteriorating.

"So you think him ill?" His lordship asked.

"O'Meara's and Stokoe's reports agree on that."

"And what do they think about the complaint in Rome?"

"They're worried about the climate and expect the worst."

"Seriously?"

"Undoubtedly."

"Well, calm your fears," Bathurst was reassuring. "I have just received intelligence that he is perfectly well."

This was said with an air of such truthfulness that Antommarchi could not contain his emotion and, seeing this, Bathurst continued: "He complains bitterly, but he has everything he could need. Government supplies him with everything he wants; indeed, he is costing us vast sums of money! However, you will soon be able to judge for yourself whether or not I tell the truth." Lowe's reports were having just the effect he hoped for – and Bathurst was falling for them!

Although he wished he could believe the intelligence report, Antommarchi was taking no chances and decided to consult the leading London physicians, especially those with tropical experience. All he approached were pleased to offer their opinions and take part in a group discussion.

"We have deliberated upon the written and verbal statements of Doctors O'Meara and Stokoe and believe that the disease affecting Napoleon is *chronic hepatitis*," was the conclusion. "This disorder almost always results from acute hepatitis, particularly when the patient, born in another country, accustomed to other climates, is obliged to live in the tropics; but it is also sometimes produced by local circumstances which have a tendency to disturb perspiration. Such is the case in the present instance.... We can affirm that the tendency to scurvy does not exist...." They did not believe that there was such a thing as an inborn predisposition to scurvy, and in this regard, they contradicted the Rome panel.

The therapeutic aspects were dealt with separately by an eminent physician who wrote to Antommarchi recommending mercurial preparations as the only means by which a radical cure could be effected. Unfortunately, he remains anonymous as he signed his letter simply 'S'. He wrote: "I should not, however, wish it to be understood that I mean to exclude all other remedies, such as local bleeding, blisters, purgatives, refrigerants, &."

Of interest, so far as Antommarchi's reputation is concerned, he added: "I am afraid you will think I am entering into superfluous details with you – who as a pupil of Mascagni must know better than anybody, that nothing so satisfactorily demonstrates the state of an organ as the manner in which it performs its functions – if I add a comment. Since the ordinary action of the mercurial medicines is to stimulate the liver to perform its natural secretions, it follows that the quantity and quality of the preparation must be adjusted to achieve that end." Antommarchi must use his experience to decide on the correct dose. As well as giving him this advice, Dr S took Antommarchi round London to a variety of establishments where he was able to demonstrate the beneficial effects of mercury on patients with chronic hepatitis acquired in India or the tropics. It was as if the name of Napoleon was an open sesame to every medical establishment, every museum and collection in town. But Antommarchi was also enjoying the status of a celebrity in the light reflected from Mascagni's great anatomical atlas – he had brought with him thirty of the plates and the proofs of the *Prodromo* (introductory volume) which had been published under the patronage of the Prince Regent; the publishers had instructed him to take advantage of the situation and present the dedication to his Royal Highness. This was satisfactorily arranged by Lord Bathurst.

On the verge of departure, events took a nasty turn. Hitherto the English police had shown no interest in Antommarchi or his activities, but when they realized he intended taking the plates with him, these suddenly became suspicious documents which he was forbidden to take to St Helena. Not to be outdone, he took them along to his lordship's office and after an hour came away with the assurance that they and a number of other books needed to complete the work would be allowed to travel with him. His lordship was not a complete Goth. But joy was short-lived.

It was not just the plates that had upset the police. There was a concerted attempt to stop Antommarchi himself going to St Helena at all, so strong were the suspicions that he was up to no good – Napoleon was not ill, and anyway there was a perfectly competent army doctor living on the spot in Longwood. He was bribed, threatened and insulted but to no avail. Two days before the party was due to leave, Antommarchi had been to take leave of some friends and was escorting a lady to her home when he was accosted by a group of men who swore at him, insulted him and abused the French in the ripest of terms. He managed to control himself, but when they included the lady in their abuse he lost his temper and would have hit out if she hadn't laid a restraining hand on his arm and steered him to the nearby home of the chief magistrate, a friend of hers.

"You were lucky our mutual friend realized what was happening," said the magistrate when the reason for their sudden call was explained, "otherwise you would have fallen into their trap and started a brawl. You would then have been arrested and detained long enough for your boat to have sailed. They were police agents."

So it was with considerable relief that Antommarchi was able to report to Gravesend, ready to sail on July 10. But when he saw the *Snipe*, her captain and crew, he felt sure they must all be part and parcel of the same conspiracy. Suspecting the worst, and much to the captain's displeasure as he swore his ship was well provisioned, Antommarchi went ashore and purchased extra supplies. And the expedition's treasurer, Abbé Buonavita wasn't too happy either. However, Antommarchi's foresightedness was justified at the first dinner when a chicken, some salt beef and a pot of beer, which would hardly have satisfied a single sailor, had to do for all six passengers. An omen that boded ill for the voyage ahead.

* * *

And now, *mon ami(e)*, you will understand that Dr Antommarchi was tarred with the Napoleonic brush. He may have been going to St Helena to take care of Napoleon but the authorities in Rome and England strongly suspected that the real reason was to investigate the possibility of Napoleon's escape.

~20~
Antommarchi is accepted into the Emperor's service

(SEPTEMBER, 1819)

With St Helena in view, the one desire of all on board was to set foot on dry land. But the cruising British warships signalled the *Snipe* forbidding her to anchor until the next morning. Anxious to learn about his patient, Antommarchi enquired how Napoleon was faring and was told, "Very well. He enjoys excellent health; he is better than we are!" Lowe's propaganda machine was in fine fettle, too!

Before the party was allowed to land, naval officers were sent on board to examine and search everyone, passengers and crew. Despite this, seventeen sealed volumes of a religious work delivered at Deptford and addressed to different people on the island, escaped detection. Judging from their size, Antommarchi guessed that they were not in fact biblical, but he didn't regard it as his responsibility to stop the captain when the books were unpacked one at a time and sent ashore.

Happily ashore, the members of the expedition were conducted to the Castle where they were astonished at the politeness of their reception. Sir Hudson introduced them to Reade and Gorrequer and to everyone else in the building at the time. He was attentive and affable and appeared to show a lively interest in the details of their voyage. Verling's appearance on the scene interrupted proceedings and when he was introduced Antommarchi thought he must have succeeded Stokoe.

"And how is Napoleon?" he asked.

"Napoleon, ..." Verling began, obviously embarrassed and

looking to the Governor for help. Lowe obliged. "Dr Verling does not attend General Bonaparte, only General Montholon."

Verling took the hint and withdrew. He told me later that he thought Antommarchi to be "rather a gentleman-like man, mild and talkative." On the other hand, Balmain, who met Antommarchi ten days later, described him as a "subtle and clever Corsican."

With Verling gone, the Governor launched into a eulogy on St Helena. What was there unpleasant about the island? The climate was good, the air healthy and the temperature tolerable, ranging between 65 and 90 degrees Fahrenheit, with no more than eight or ten degrees variation between Longwood and Jamestown. Typical, thought Antommarchi remembering what O'Meara had told him about the Governor. The introduction at last at an end, the new arrivals were invited to dine at Plantation House.

Over the meal the Governor and his immediate staff were excessively polite and attentive – Lowe had to get the doctor on side. But when Antommarchi asked about Napoleon he set the Governor off on his usual rant, blaming the General's pride and stubbornness for all his difficulties and complaining bitterly about some of the protests he had made – as Governor he deserved to be more respectfully treated.

Dinner over, and before the new arrivals were allowed to leave they had to submit to yet another inspection. After sincere apologies Major Gorrequer made them empty their pockets and open their pocket-books. Reade, who was much more thorough, opened and examined every article in their possession.

Once on their way Antommarchi could appreciate St Helena for what it really was: "Wherever we looked we saw nothing but sentries and precipices; on one side a deep abyss, on the other a fierce-looking soldier. We proceeded thus amidst the precautions of war and the convulsions of nature, and never before had we seen so gloomy a spectacle." Welcome to Longwood!

On their arrival, Napoleon was closeted with Bertrand reading a copy of the *Morning Chronicle* which had just arrived from London. It spoke of Antommarchi, praising him as an anatomist but said not a word about Antommarchi the physician. What on earth was the Cardinal up to? Had he, perhaps, had some intimation from above? Napoleon told Bertrand to find out just what sort of man the Cardinal had sent.

Bertrand first took Buonavita in to Napoleon. After a while he came out and led Antommarchi to another room where he proceeded to subject him to a thorough interrogation: Had he met the Emperor's family? How were they? Why had he been chosen as Napoleon's physician? In what capacity had he been sent? Had he any letter or document for Napoleon from his family? (The lack of these was something that had deeply troubled Antommarchi from the start, particularly the absence of an introductory letter from Cardinal Fesch.) Who had he met on the journey?

With these questions answered to Bertrand's satisfaction, Antommarchi was introduced to Madame Bertrand who was socializing with Verling and Buonavita. After supper he was shown his room. He had just started to undress when Bertrand knocked at the door and told him that Montholon wanted to see him again. Utterly perplexed, he wondered what more he could possibly be asked – and at that hour, too. But all Montholon wanted to know was his motive for coming to St Helena? That, he could easily answer: An ambition to serve the Emperor, the greatest man of the age – and he wasn't being sycophantic.

When he got back to his room, the reason for the lateness of the summons, Jacques Chandelier, the chef, was waiting outside in the ante-chamber. He wanted to know if he could sleep there. His interview with Montholon had gone on late and he had not yet been assigned a room. He thought Antommarchi would be interested that both he and Coursot had already seen the Emperor who wanted to know what had been said in Rome regarding the choice of physician and priests; what they had seen and heard about them in London; what houses they had visited there? It now became all too apparent to Antommarchi that he had aroused the suspicion and mistrust of the French – as if it wasn't bad enough being suspected and mistrusted by the English. Did no one trust him? The next morning, the twenty-first, he had a third visit from Bertrand who asked him to write out a comprehensive curriculum vitae with particular attention to where and for long he had practised, whether he had been attached to any service and whether he devoted himself to any branch of the profession. This he did immediately and sent the result to Bertrand with his diplomas, papers and the letter of December 19 from Cardinal Fesch appointing him to the post. Both Buonavita and Vignali had also had to compile their life stories.

Actually, it was no wonder they were under suspicion. They had been sent by the British Government, recommended by Lord Bathurst (Napoleon's blackest *bête noir* outside the island) and graciously received by the Governor. Added to this was the absence of any letter from a member of the Emperor's family – and not only had the Cardinal failed to send a letter of introduction, he had even tried to get Vignali recognized as Napoleon's physician. Indeed, Fesch had written to Las Cases asking him to recommend Vignali as such to the Emperor – this was without doubt an attempt by the Church to gain access to Napoleon's body as well as his soul. But Las Cases didn't think it proper to transform a priest into a physician. He simply passed the Cardinal's letter on to Buonavita.

Eventually, Napoleon accepted that they were who they said they were, Frenchmen and Corsicans, and not agents for the British. He accepted them into his service.

With this settled, on the twenty-second Antommarchi set off on his own to collect his baggage which was still on board the *Snipe*. Although he had been assured by the Governor that he would be free to go wherever he wished, he was nevertheless intercepted by Captain Nicholls who was under orders to accompany him. To his surprise he found the ship's captain in a similar situation: he had been stopped going ashore to sell his goods and was raging around his ship in a right paddy. And the crime he had committed? The supposed religious pamphlets had turned out to be nothing of the kind. They were copies of the tract O'Meara had written against the Governor: *An Exposition of some of the Transactions that have Taken Place at St. Helena, since the Appointment of Sir Hudson Lowe as Governor of that Island* (1819). It was a wonder the captain hadn't been placed under arrest.

Back at Longwood, Antommarchi was given a letter from Bertrand:

"The Emperor accepts you as his surgeon, and allows you a salary of nine thousand francs a year. Your duties will start as soon as you have taken the oath...."

The oath amounted to agreeing not to communicate with, or say anything to, the English, and to take special care not to give them the least information about the progress of the Emperor's disorder. Since all he had experienced and heard about the English had taught him the sort of people he had to deal with, Antommarchi had no hesitation in taking the oath.

The time had now arrived for him to be presented to his new employer.

* * *

And now, *mon ami(e)*, you will understand that after long months without medical attention Napoleon once again has a personal physician – and, despite attempts to denigrate him, he was an excellent and well-qualified doctor anxious to serve his Emperor. Without question Napoleon was a sick man, suffering from hepatitis (endemic on the island) and cholecystitis (though that was not yet recognized as a disease in its own right). His health fluctuated and he enjoyed periods of reasonable well-being. And remember that the British still stubbornly refuse to accept that he suffered from ill-health at all, a view bolstered by the Governor's fabricated bulletins.

~21~
'Let medicine command"!

The room was small and very gloomy. At first Antommarchi had difficulty making out the figure of Napoleon lying in bed. He groped his way forward, quietly and with a sense almost of religious awe, until he heard Napoleon say in a friendly voice, "*Approach, Capo Corsinaccio*, so that I can see you better and hear you better; I have become quite deaf living on this miserable rock." He spoke in Italian, the language he was always to use when they spoke together.

And so began a long, long conversation that was more in the nature of an interrogation. Napoleon was desperate to suck Antommarchi dry of every last drop of news and information about his old world. With his usual charm he first put his new doctor at ease with talk of Corsica, before moving on to the details of his career and his motives for exchanging the culture of Florence for the iniquity that was St Helena; he needed to hear the answers from Antommarchi himself, not at second-hand from Bertrand. And what of Fesch's letter to Las Cases attempting to have Vignali accepted as sole physician? This had seriously annoyed him. What, for heaven's sake, was Fesch up to? He sent me an anatomist when I had asked for a physician. And then he has second thoughts; he is more concerned with collecting souls than with my health in this world.

Napoleon proceeded to extract everything Antommarchi knew about the members of the imperial family, before reaching the grand finale of an in-depth grilling on his stay in Rome and the journey to London.

When Antommarchi was eventually dismissed he was told to see Verling and ask who he was looking after and the treatment he was prescribing; and while he was at it, what were the prevalent diseases on the island, particularly at Longwood:

"This island is quite another world; you require the advice of those who have studied it. Although I have constantly refused to see your predecessor, I nevertheless think he can give you all the information you need to succeed here in the exercise of your profession. Try to persuade him to remain a few days longer so that you may discover all the information that may be essential to you." Here we have a clear indication of the depth of the Emperor's stubbornness in refusing to consult Verling, no matter how ill he was.

But Napoleon was not finished with Antommarchi. An hour or two later the doctor was again summoned. This time the Emperor was in the drawing-room, lit only by a single candle. Napoleon took him by the ears, laughing, and then the questioning began again, mostly to clarify some of the answers from the first time round. Napoleon next put Antommarchi through a rigorous examination all the while displaying a remarkable knowledge of anatomy and physiology. This completed to the Emperor's satisfaction, he was told to go to bed.

Antommarchi visited his patient in a professional capacity for the first time on September 23 and, for a change, in a room sufficiently well lit to allow him to make an adequate examination. Napoleon was lying on his camp bed; he was, as he had said, hard of hearing – possibly the consequence of a lifetime's exposure to artillery fire, particularly in his early years as an artillery officer.

It was a very unhealthy man who confronted Antommarchi. His complexion was ghastly with its black rings around eyes that were bloodshot and tinged with jaundice. His tongue had a whitish coating and his nostrils were discoloured and blocked. He had been off his food for several days, complaining of nausea and vomiting.

In response to Antommarchi's questions, he said that there was nothing amiss with his micturition apart from frequency and difficulty in starting, which he had been cursed with since childhood. He did, however, complain of vague pains in his right side and more particularly of a pain in the right upper part of his abdomen which varied in intensity and had been present for a long time; Napoleon tried to identify its precise location by saying it felt about two inches below the surface. He also complained of a fairly constant, moderately acute pain in the region of the right breast and of a sensation of extreme discomfort in his right shoulder. Every day, he said, he had episodes of profuse sweating.

The patient Antommarchi then proceeded to examine had an excessively fat body, a very pale skin and a pulse that was regular at a rate of about 60 per minute. He said he could feel the left lobe of his liver in the central region of the upper abdomen; it was hard and when he pressed it, extremely tender. He said he was also able to feel the gall-bladder under the rib margin on the right side; it was full and firm. The diagnosis of chronic hepatitis made by both O'Meara and Stokoe was thus confirmed.

The whole time he was being examined, Napoleon didn't stop talking:

"I like your frankness, your independent spirit," he began, "you have given up everything to come and attend me – it is only right that I should also do something by way of return. I therefore resign myself; let medicine command, I submit to its decisions and entrust my health to your hands." (Where have we heard that before?)

Next morning at a quarter past ten Antommarchi was initiated into the daily routine that had been O'Meara's for nearly three years. The Emperor was still in bed after a bad night, complaining of vague pains, particularly in the right breast. Antommarchi advised a bath, a sedative medicine and massage with an ammonia and opium liniment. By half-past two his patient was better and ready to talk.

"I understand you have published the posthumous works of Mascagni; I should very much like to see the plates as the English papers have spoken so highly of them."

They did indeed greatly impress the Emperor.

"But you know, doctor," he said, "you have upset all my previous ideas; I am at a loss to know what to make of your work. Your *Prodromo* is a revolution in anatomy. You mercilessly criticize everything that has been written on the subject."

"I believe so, Sire, for it corrects many findings wrongly arrived at."

"And does not contain any opinions too lightly arrived at?"

"I believe not."

"But your teaching is totally different from the way we teach in our schools. What will the anatomists say when they see their old and accepted theories so demolished?"

What indeed!

As Antommarchi was taking his leave: "Two hours of anatomy for a man who never could bear the sight of a dead body!" said the man who had seen many thousands and been responsible for the creation of many more. "Ah! doctor, what are you thinking about? You are a seducer; you will soon persuade me that pills are pleasant things to take."

Napoleon's next bout of vague pains in the abdomen were soon relieved by an enema. Afterwards, still seated on the commode, he admitted he had not been out of the house for eighteen months. Antommarchi insisted that for the sake of his general health it was essential that he get outside and take some exercise. Napoleon submitted and by October 3, the two were taking regular morning walks in the garden after he had had his bath. Nevertheless, Napoleon still refused to consider Antommarchi's recommendation of mercury, whether internally or externally. So much for "let medicine command, I submit to its decisions and entrust my health to your hands." He was still the same old Napoleon!

This state of affairs continued until the end of the year with episodes of mild abdominal pain, sometimes accompanied by a headache or gloomy dejection, which were relieved by baths or enemas. There was also a handful of more acute and 'violent' pains in the liver which responded within a day or two to the same measures.

Aware that Napoleon was never going to make a full recovery unless he was moved from Longwood (and preferably from the island), Antommarchi constantly complained to the Governor about the unhealthy conditions on the plateau. And as constantly Lowe contradicted him. Longwood, he said, enjoyed the healthiest climate he knew on the island and that was precisely why it had been chosen.

However, anxious that Antommarchi should make up his own mind about conditions on the island, Napoleon told him to write to the Governor for permission to visit the local hospitals. Permission was granted but only on condition he was accompanied by a British officer: "A most prudent precaution! So warlike an individual as myself might stir the sick into sedition and beat England with a few dying patients!"

The visit took place on October 10. "I am well and do not require any doctoring today," said Napoleon. "Go and take advantage of the *Sicilian*'s permission to visit the hospitals. In fact," he said, looking out of the window, "I think I see one of his *Kalmoucks* coming; probably the one appointed to watch over you."

Napoleon had guessed correctly and the '*Kalmouck*' turned out to be Dr Archibald Arnott, surgeon to the 20th Regiment. Their first port of call was the military hospital in Jamestown where Antommarchi saw almost nothing but 'dysentery' and acute and chronic hepatitis; a few patients had 'inflammatory fevers'. He saw nothing he had not got at Longwood.

The military hospital at Deadwood camp was a different matter. Although it displayed much the same disorders as those he had seen in Jamestown, their progress was much more rapid. So much so that patients could be beyond help within an hour of admission.

Next morning, a sarcastic Napoleon greeted Antommarchi and his report: "You are an ignoramus, Sir," he began. "Bathurst would even say a dishonest man, a traitor! Liver complaints! Why they are unknown on the island. Ask the Governor, the minister, ask all England. This is the most salubrious spot on the globe! Do you not know that hepatitis is not tolerated on St. Helena? That man, Sir Hudson, will not admit those kinds of disorders; he forbids them even to approach the shoreline, though every other disease has permission to put in here.

"A little while ago Madame Montholon thought there could be no harm in suffering from a disease she had already suffered in Paris. She asked to be allowed to return to Europe but was told it was all in her imagination – and her doctor [Verling] was severely reprimanded. He soon acknowledged his error, and the seat of the complaint was removed to some other place. It was no longer the liver that was affected, but another organ, I forget which, and that alone. His Excellency then assented, and granted a passage. Ah! doctor, what men we have to deal with!"

Had Antommarchi made his inspection a week or two later, however, he would have been presented with the picture that Balmain sent to the Tsar on November 5: "The spring equinox has again brought us its toll of dysentery, liver troubles, and inflammatory fevers. The great hospital in town is filled with patients from the 20th Regiment." And again on the twenty-sixth: "The number of sick, especially among the soldiers of the 20th, is increasing every day. The average is twenty per company (of sixty men). It is a kind of grippe, which has come upon us suddenly and affects principally the liver or the abdomen. The Admiral (Plampin) has had all the convalescent men of his squadron taken up to a hilltop, where the fresher air contributes to their complete recovery. Captain de Gors has been dangerously ill. I myself have been suffering for five weeks from my liver."

* * *

And now, *mon ami(e)*, you will appreciate that Antommarchi began his attendance on a very unhealthy emperor who had not been out of doors for eighteen months. Although he was suffering from chronic hepatitis, cholecystitis with biliary colic (from gallstones), and conceivably something going on in the region of his stomach, you must view these against a background of a prolonged unhealthy lifestyle, loss of freedom, shocking living conditions, unfavourable climate with its endemic diseases, poor nutrition and constant mental stress all of which conspired to lower his resistance to disease.

~22~

"Come, we must cultivate our garden"

(NOVEMBER, 1819 – JULY, 1820)

An unexpected by-product of the arrival of the two missionaries was the cause of much grief to the Governor. Whenever his soldiers met them, they would run and kneel before them. And no sooner did the Irishmen among them see the cassock than they would prostrate themselves, kiss their hands and feet and beg for benediction. The Governor, for some reason, blamed the missionaries themselves and had them closely watched. So far as the troops were concerned, he resorted to increased supervision, reprimands or outright punishment, but piety prevailed over fear and holy water over flogging. Napoleon, for his part, could not see why Lowe attached such importance to the exchange of a few genuflexions and 'Hail Marys', but what really upset him was the manner in which the missionaries were being treated.

"I shall not allow that heretic to humble St Peter's halo," he said with a laugh. "If I were to let these insults pass unnoticed, the Pope and Consistory would never forgive me." He then called Buonavita and ordered him not to venture beyond the Longwood limits again. "Let people say, after that, that I do not take care to see that the Church is respected."

During his morning walk with Antommarchi on November 16, a gloomy Napoleon began asking questions about his symptoms. He had been worrying about his father's last illness which had been attributed to cancer of the stomach. Was he suffering from the same condition?

Carlo Bonaparte, he said, was already ill when, at the beginning of 1785, he took his eldest daughter to school in Paris. He was losing weight and suffering badly with indigestion. Suspecting his days were numbered, he started home, but only got as far as Montpellier when he began to vomit almost continuously. Physicians and their medicines could do nothing for him until someone advised him to follow a particular diet and to eat juicy pears. So he returned to Paris where pears were more plentiful and of better quality. He ate a massive number, took a lot of exercise, recovered and returned to Corsica, fit and active with the complexion of a man "likely to live two hundred years." Regrettably, it was only a remission and he had not been home for long before he was worse than ever. Since the advice he had been given at Montpellier had proved life saving, he decided to return in the hope that they might be able to repeat the performance. But his hour had come, no medicine could help and he died at the age of thirty-nine.

"The Montpellier doctors believed there was something unusual about his complaint, so they opened him up to find a 'scirrhus at the pylorus'." (If you ask me this was most likely to have been a duodenal ulcer.)

"Do you think that kind of affection can be transmitted with the gift of life?" Napoleon asked.

"No, Sire; diseases no more pass from father to son than dispositions and talents."

On the eighteenth Napoleon was quite well again though complaining of the lassitude born of inactivity.

"What am I to do, doctor?"

"Take some exercise."

"Where?"

" In the garden. In the park. Anywhere in the open air."

"What! In the middle of the redcoats?"

"No, Sire. You must dig and so escape from inactivity and insult at the same time."

"Dig! Yes, doctor, you are right, I *shall* dig."

He began work early the next morning. He appointed Noverraz, a countryman, as head gardener to work under his direction, and together they had already turned over a sizeable plot of land when Antommarchi arrived to see what had been achieved.

"Well, doctor, are you pleased with your patient?" He held up his spade. "This is better than your pills; you shall not physic me any more. Come, we must cultivate our garden." So saying he set to work again but, after a few minutes, he stopped:

"This is too much like hard work; I'm exhausted and my hands are sore. Another time." And he threw down the spade. "You are laughing. Never mind, I have always made my body bend to my will, and it shall do so again."

As good as his word, he quickly grew fond of his self-appointed task, though not so the male inhabitants of Longwood who were all cajoled into service.

Soon the garden was transformed. Ponds and waterfalls, paths and grottoes were created, willows and oaks and peaches planted. The garden became a living thing. Once the ornamental side was completed, Napoleon turned his attention to the useful. He divided the land into allotments which he and his labourers trenched and manured before sowing with beans and peas and every other vegetable that would grow on the island.

When the Governor came to hear of all this activity he, inevitably, suspected it was cover for a conspiracy. Arriving to investigate, he asked Antommarchi, "Is it on your advice that General Bonaparte is indulging in this violent exercise?"

Yes it was, Antommarchi replied, which puzzled the Governor. He shrugged his shoulders: "You work yourselves to death by transplanting trees in a waterless soil under a merciless sun; it is pointless labour, everything dies, nothing will survive." Could Lowe have forgotten that he had described Longwood as enjoying the healthiest climate he knew on the island?

Antommarchi politely thanked the Governor for his solicitude and assured him he had too unfavourable an opinion of the country under his command: "The young shoots are doing very well and many are already in bud." When Antommarchi told Napoleon of the encounter, the response was predictable: "The wretch is jealous of every minute he is unable to poison me."

By the time Christmas was on the horizon, Napoleon had enjoyed a month of uninterrupted good health with his digestive system working well. He spent his days happily gardening, walking and talking about anything that happened to crop up; but on the seventeenth of December all this shuddered to a halt. His disorder vigorously reasserted itself – acute pains of biliary colic, with all the symptoms of an inflammation of the bowels. Antommarchi prescribed the usual bath, simple enemas and soothing fomentations on the abdomen. He also recommended castor oil.

Next day the pains were less severe but still Napoleon could not rest comfortably. He developed a dry, painful cough which, however, responded to calming medicines. By the evening of the nineteenth the Emperor was feeling better; the biliary colic had completely disappeared and his bowels had settled.

The improvement continued and on the twenty-first he went out for a short walk. Antommarchi had also been out and when he got home he called on Napoleon who was surprised to see him; he thought he was showing a party of English physicians round the grounds. (Despite Napoleon no longer receiving visitors, travellers who had the Governor's permission could still visit Longwood.) Antommarchi explained that individually they had all been looking forward to the visit, but at the last moment, acting as a group, they had sent an apology. "I don't know whether the hand that kept them back may not be the same that has just caused me to be arrested." Returning from his evening constitutional in the park he had been stopped by the sentry at the Longwood gate and taken to the guardroom. He was released after a few minutes.

The same thing happened a few days later, only this time he was kept in the guardroom for half-an-hour and regained his liberty only on the arrival of the sergeant of the guard. Napoleon was incensed at this and suggested he write to the Governor and say he would leave the island if this harassment continued.

Antommarchi did just that and, as was the habit of the times, at great length, detailing all the circumstances. Napoleon read the letter and, no doubt anticipating Lowe's response, told him also to write to Hamilton (the Earl of Aberdeen – a force to be reckoned with in political and diplomatic circles) who had taken an interest in Antommarchi and had praised his work. This he did, at even greater length and adorned with purple patches:

"….Although my time is devoted to study and the relief of suffering humanity on this island, which nature seems to have stamped with a deep impression of melancholy and rejection, I see all its inhabitants shun the neighbourhood of Longwood with as much dread as, in eternity, they might fly from the approach to Hell. This terror seems to have taken possession of their minds, to the total exclusion of every other feeling."

He complained that his professional colleagues would have little or nothing to do with him since the least word or contact would be reported to the Governor. He continued with a particularly revealing observation:

"Telescopes, directed at our houses, pry into our apartments, and telegraphs, very cunningly contrived, instantly report everything that takes place inside." And further on, "If I wish to stray beyond the narrow limits within which we are confined, I am obliged to accept the company of one of the governor's agents who is under instructions to give him a faithful account of everything I may do or say in his presence."

Eventually he reached the *raison d'être* of the letter which he presented clearly and with commendable succinctness. He ended with hope that Hamilton's mediation with Lord Bathurst "will have the effect of rendering my residence on this island less melancholy and less unpleasant."

And this it did! While the letter to the Governor influenced him little or not at all, that to Hamilton moved mountains: "The limits were widened and I could henceforth breathe and circulate freely, and had no longer to fear being taken to the guardroom, or wounded by the thrust of a bayonet." Lowe was overwhelmed to the extent that he even agreed to Antommarchi's request not to intercept his letters. "This solicitude was most affecting, but very ill-bestowed."

Napoleon then thought he would amuse himself at the suitably chastened Governor's expense. He was digging a new pond and turned up for work dressed like one of the Chinese in a large pair of trousers and jacket with an enormous straw hat on his head and sandals on his feet. Together, he and Antommarchi walked towards a group of Chinese workmen. As they approached, the Chinese stared at the antics of these strange foreigners, giggling with half-suppressed merriment. After digging with them for a while, Napoleon disappeared, returning almost immediately on horseback accompanied by his groom. He rode up and down for a few minutes before suddenly taking off at a gallop towards Deadwood. On reaching the high point, he stopped, scanned the land around through his telescope, and rode back as quickly as he had come.

This fairly put the cat among the Governor's pigeons. The telegraphs were humming. A horseman had been seen, dressed like a Chinese. Who was he? Where had he come from? What was he doing? The Governor was as desperate as Napoleon guessed he would be. So, to stick a pin in the cat's behind, Napoleon enlisted the help of the young Abbé Vignali, dressed him in Chinese clothes similar to those he himself was wearing, sat him on his horse, gave him his telescope and his groom and told him to ride fast and appear to be making observations. The whole island was in an uproar. Lowe, Gorrequer and Reade appeared at Longwood in an instant. What was going on? Only Vignali indulging himself. The Governor, now even more confused, left.

On his way out he intercepted Antommarchi who made a convenient target for his pent-up anger. He ended his outburst by declaring that the person who laughed at his expense was only a usurper who had wrongfully claimed power and victories.

"No doubt!" Antommarchi innocently replied.

Taken aback, a thoroughly perplexed Governor invited Antommarchi to speak freely, hoping to get to the bottom of this unexpected concession.

"The Emperor – for by calling him General, you acquit him of one of his usurpations, and I want to reckon them all – is indeed guilty many times over of the crime of which you accuse him." And so Antommarchi launched into a catalogue of all the Emperor's victories and triumphs. He had reached the Egyptian campaign, when Lowe decided he had heard enough and made his escape.

"Well, what did Hudson say? Is he afraid that some day I shall sprout wings, take flight and escape the grave?"

"I know not, Sire. I was telling him how you had usurped victory and public admiration; the sketch displeased him."

Although pleasantly amused, Napoleon felt the Governor had been baited enough for one day and turned his attention back to the task in hand.

For the first six months of 1820 the General and his team of landscaping artists made excellent progress with the digging of ponds and laying of pipes to bring their water from close on three-quarters of a mile away.

On July 7 a little cheer went up as the first tentative gushes of water left the pipe. "This is good," said the Emperor, "but where shall we put the aviary?" One job completed, his mind immediately turned to the next.

"Here, Sire?"

"No, further behind you; it will be better there; it's a more open aspect. You will arrange that, doctor, so long as nothing serious prevents it."

As if on cue, Napoleon's disorder, which Antommarchi had considered, if not completely resolved, at least considerably abated, suddenly relapsed and with a vengeance.

* * *

And now, *mon ami(e)*, you understand why O'Meara, Stokoe and Antommarchi, each in turn, were so insistent that Napoleon took plenty of exercise in the fresh air. By getting him to take fairly vigorous exercise in the form of landscape gardening, Antommarchi achieved the almost impossible; in just over a year he transformed Napoleon's existence on the island.

But alas, it couldn't last.

~23~
The last picnic

(JULY – OCTOBER, 1820)

Napoleon had enjoyed the seven months of autumn and early winter in good health, taking plenty of exercise and delighting in his active supervision of the gardening project. All was going well, to an extent that had not been seen at Longwood for quite some time. However, on July 7 he suffered a relapse that seriously worried Antommarchi. So seriously, in fact, that he felt the imperial family should be kept informed. Accordingly, he obtained Napoleon's permission to write to the Chevalier Colonna in Rome:

"The Emperor has recently had a most serious relapse – burning fever, deep and severe pain in the liver; acute pulsating pain in the right ankle joint with an erysipelatous inflammation extending along the dorsum of the foot and a third of the way up the front of the leg," he wrote on the eighteenth. "I do not hesitate to say that these afflictions are caused by a disordered state of the digestive system and an alteration of the function of the biliary organs. The patient's case does not, however, present any imminent danger, but precludes all hope of recovery in a tropical climate. Little by little the morbid signs spread and grow more serious, and I am afraid my help and my prayers may soon be as cruelly dashed as your hopes."

In case you're wondering, erysipelas is an acute streptococcal infection of the skin. The inflammatory rash is usually accompanied by chills, fever and sometimes nausea and vomiting. However, Antommarchi should have held back from saying that the erysipelas was caused by the abdominal disorders because it would have been the other way round.

The illness reached its height about a fortnight later when, in addition to the symptoms of erysipelas, in particular a swollen and very painful right lower leg and foot, Napoleon complained of an exceptionally severe pain in the liver which extended into the shoulder, making his breathing difficult and painful. Antommarchi ordered rest, cold refreshing drinks, local fomentations, soapy liniments and the ubiquitous enema.

This relapse, which was, as I said, a response to the continuing erysipelas, pursued an up-and-down course for another ten days at the end of which the Emperor's skin was tinged with jaundice. But by the end of the month all was well again and Napoleon was once more enjoying the delights of his garden.

Although he felt well throughout August and the first fortnight of September, it was too good to last: the pain in the liver returned with increased severity; he lost his appetite and suffered with bilious vomiting. He felt exhausted at the mere thought of going for a walk. Moreover, he was beginning to live in the past.

When Antommarchi made his visit on the eighteenth of September he was greeted by a bed-ridden patient with sunken eyes; jaundiced conjunctivae and skin; a green tinge to his complexion and a whitish coating to his tongue. Pressure over the upper centre part of his abdomen was painful. His breathing was difficult with intermittent deep sighs. At 80 beats per minute his pulse was raised above his normal rate of around 60. After much persuasion, Antommarchi managed to get his patient to take a dose of a cholagogue (a purgative that empties the gall-bladder into the duodenum) which brought great relief.

Incidentally, the green tinge to Napoleon's complexion is an intriguing observation. The fact that it was sufficiently evident for Antommarchi to record, suggests that it should be given more than a mere passing glance. A green tinge to the skin is a sign of chlorosis, now known to be caused by iron-deficiency anaemia. Chlorosis, the green sickness or the disease of virgins (it occurred most frequently in serving girls at the onset of menstruation), was once extremely common but is now rare, probably owing to improved living conditions despite the fact that iron-deficiency anaemia is still very much with us. If the green tinge to Napoleon's complexion was indeed attributable to iron-deficiency anaemia – and considering the circumstances of his existence on St Helena, this would certainly come as no surprise – a number of his less ominous symptoms, such as tiredness, lack of energy, breathlessness on exertion, swelling of the ankles, could be attributed, in whole or certainly in part, to the deficiency. Whether it contributed to the progress of Napoleon's main diseases is anybody's guess, though it would certainly have done them no good.

A pointer to the diagnosis of cholecystitis with gallstones is the relief he obtained from the cholagogue, indicating that the medicine had probably expelled one or more gallstones from the biliary tract. The difficulty with his breathing, on the other hand, is more worrying as it could have been a sign of heart failure.

The symptoms varied in intensity over the next few days, occasionally easing to the extent that on the twentieth Napoleon was tempted to go for a drive in his carriage but after a few minutes was so overcome by fatigue that he had to return. He rejected every treatment Antommarchi had to offer – tonics, raising blisters on the arm and nape of the neck and, especially, the opening of an issue in the left arm – both these last showing medicine's continued adherence to some aspects of the ancient doctrine of the humours. He did, however, persist in his attempts at outdoor exercise, though without success until October 4.

Early that morning Napoleon set out with all his usual attendants for a picnic wherever the spirit might lead them. Napoleon alternated between horseback and carriage, but he was being far too ambitious. After five-and-a-half miles the expedition arrived on the northern lip of the Great Crater overlooking Sandy Bay towards the Atlantic Ocean.

"I must rest." He had had enough.

By accident or design, Mount Pleasant, home of Sir William Doveton, a prominent member of the island Council, was only a short distance away and thither Montholon was sent to present the Emperor's compliments and might he come and rest himself? Sir William was only too pleased to put his home at the Emperor's disposal and invited him to join the family inside. With Bertrand's help, Napoleon made it up the steps to the drawing-room and the welcoming haven of the sofa.

He immediately began talking to his host, a slow process as Sir William did not speak French and everything had to be conducted through Bertrand whose command of English was only adequate. In due course, Sir William asked whether the Emperor would join him for breakfast, but Napoleon declined saying they had brought their own picnic and would like to take it on the lawn. While Montholon prepared the table outside, Napoleon stayed indoors to meet the other members of the Doveton family, making quite a hit with the children who all were given little pieces of liquorice from a tortoiseshell box.

When the picnic breakfast was ready, Sir William joined them at Napoleon's request, bringing with him a pint bottle of Mount Pleasant water, a local rot-gut potion otherwise known as orange shrub (an orange cordial reinforced with sugar, spices and a spirit, usually rum). The meal finished, Napoleon filled a small tumbler with champagne for Sir William and another for himself. Then another and another and a final glass of shrub. Back indoors he resumed his seat on the sofa until he decided it was time to head off back to Longwood.

He reached Longwood at two in the afternoon, went straight to his bedroom and, leaving instructions not to be disturbed, flung himself down on his bed utterly exhausted – and no wonder!

This visit was memorable for being Napoleon's last excursion outside the imposed limits of Longwood. Its aftermath was a severe hangover to add to the existing pain in his liver which had increased and still extended to his right shoulder. He continued to complain of a troublesome heaviness and deep pain in the left side under the ribs. He was getting progressively weaker.

During the night of the twelfth he woke with a violent headache and constipation to a degree that even enemas could not dislodge. He was so weak that the slightest movement made him vertiginous. But at two in the morning his bowels opened mightily leaving him quite exhausted. This evacuation reduced the intensity of the symptoms, although at about five o'clock a new pain appeared: it extended down the line of the vertebral column from the nape of the neck and the shoulders to the middle of the back – strongly indicative of the leakage of a gastric ulcer into the peritoneal cavity.

On the fifteenth, after a quiet night, Napoleon still complained of headache, although his appetite was recovering and he started belching frequently. And at last Antommarchi persuaded the Emperor to let him apply blisters, though he might have saved himself the bother as they were virtually without effect. At 4am Napoleon was visited by another great evacuation which was, understandably, attended by violent gripings. Nevertheless, during the day, with his strength returning, he went for a two-hour walk in the garden. That night he suffered from colic and more evacuations which were beginning to contain undigested food. In the morning, feeling a bit better, he took another stroll in the garden.

His improvement continued over the next two days with both his strength and his appetite returning. Despite this, the acute pain in his left side returned, impelling him to complain to Antommarchi:

"Is there anything more deplorable than my existence here? It is not living, it is vegetating. I shall never get better. Perhaps death will soon bring an end to my sufferings." And he asked Antommarchi to carry out his post-mortem, since the last thing he wanted was for a doctor of the Governor's choice to do it.

The next time Napoleon complained of this pain, Antommarchi ill-advisedly remarked on the changes that had been taking place in the functions of the imperial stomach as well as in those of the liver.

"What are you saying about the stomach? Know, Sir, that mine is sound, and that I have never, in any place, or under any circumstances, suffered the slightest pain from it. Therefore no more on that subject; do you hear?"

The next day saw little change, but on the thirty-first Antommarchi found him lying on the sofa under several covers even though the thermometer in the room was registering 65 to 66 degrees Fahrenheit. In the course of a restless night he had had, one after another, eight evacuations of liquid, undigested faecal material and during the day he added another three to the score. His legs were almost constantly cold and as he persisted in his refusal to take any medicines, Antommarchi simply prescribed a strict diet, rice-water and enemas (to try to empty the intestines and save Napoleon the inconvenience of having to do so unaided).

And thus did October come to a close.

* * *

And now, *mon ami(e)*, you understand that, despite spells of reasonable well-being that even let him go on a picnic, Napoleon's overall health was in steady decline – helped on its way, no doubt, by the picnic! The most important disease that was announcing its arrival was a gastric ulcer.

~24~
Quod scriptum, scriptum

(NOVEMBER, 1820 – APRIL 1, 1821)

At the beginning of November, Antommarchi decided to re-introduce Napoleon to sea-water baths. Whether cause and effect or not, the improvement was impressive and Napoleon resumed his walks in the garden and his rides in the carriage – but not for long. On the eleventh/twelfth, the pain in his liver returned with increased severity and the acute pain up the spine made a reappearance, probably meaning that the sealed-off leakage from a gastric ulcer had leaked again and had again become sealed off.

Understandably, the Emperor was depressed and apathetic. On the nineteenth he confided to Antommarchi:

"What a delightful thing is rest! The bed has become a place of luxury for me; I wouldn't exchange it for all the thrones in the world. . . I, whose activity was boundless; I, whose mind never slept, am now plunged into the deepest lethargy, and must make an effort even to raise my eyelids! I sometimes dictated upon different subjects to four or five secretaries who wrote as fast as I could speak – but then I *was* Napoleon; now I am no longer anything; my strength, my faculties have deserted me; I do not live, I merely exist."

At the beginning of December he felt well enough to go for a number of rides in the carriage until, in the middle of the month, he found this too much. Even sometimes when walking about his drawing room his legs would give way and he would be compelled to sit down. And so it continued until Christmas Day which was not a merry one. His Christmas present to Antommarchi was to allow him to clean the imperial teeth, something he had resisted for a long time and which had been a significant contributor to his background ill-health.

Boxing Day looked to have benefited from the improved dental hygiene until, reading the latest newspapers to reach the island, he came across the news of his sister, Elisa's, death. It affected him badly. He was grief stricken, slumped in his armchair, utterly silent. At length he looked up and, gazing fixedly at Antommarchi, stretched out his arm, a gesture seeking comfort. But Antommarchi's instinctive reaction was to grasp his wrist and take his pulse – which he found to be weak and irregular! A drink of orange-flower water (some had been found since O'Meara's departure) induced considerable belching followed by hiccups. He risked another drink before venturing into the garden to sit on a bench.

"Ah! doctor, how tired I am! I do, though, admit that my oppression is considerably lifted. The orange-flower water has freed me from that overabundance of wind that was wearing me out. I feel the fresh air can now do me some good." Ah well!

Back indoors, he went to bed. After a while he sent for Antommarchi who found him greatly depressed with a tongue thickly coated in white matter and a mouth and throat well covered with a viscid, phlegm-like substance. Although Antommarchi hadn't commented on it in the intervening months the coating on the tongue had been present since his initial examination some eighteen months previously. You would recognize it as oral thrush, a fungal infection to which run-down patients are particularly prone.

The General's condition remained much unchanged until the thirtieth which proved to be a really bad day. Even so, he persisted in his refusal to take any medicine internally.

"Apply on the exterior every remedy you think proper, I have no objection. But to introduce into my body a mass of preparations and ingredients capable of destroying the strongest constitution, is what I will never consent to. I will not have two diseases, one given by nature, and the other by the physician." He would not be the last by any manner of means to feel that way!

When Antommarchi paid his morning visit on January 2, Napoleon was feeling better. Still in bed, he wanted some air. As Antommarchi was opening the window, it slipped and, in trying to catch it, it sliced the back of his hand. In a trice the Emperor was out of bed: "Doctor, you have cut your hand! Quick! A physician!" And to the servants: "Go and find one of the English surgeons! Wounds are dangerous here; the least delay may be fatal. Hurry, someone run to the camp [Deadwood]". When action was called for, Napoleon was still your man despite all his fatigue and depression. Antommarchi was quite affected and, indeed, confused by this display of concern; so much so that he thought more about calming the Emperor than of treating his own injury.

The wound was in fact quite serious as the extensor tendons of the last three fingers of his right hand were exposed and almost cut through. Nevertheless, he wasn't prepared to wait for help to arrive and dressed the wound himself. Not unexpectedly, he developed a fever and it was three days before he felt well enough to attend the Emperor again. During those three days Napoleon constantly asked how he was getting on.

Feeling better, Napoleon resumed his exercise in the garden and his rides in the carriage. However, his response to Antommarchi's never-ceasing pleas to take his medicines was to stick to his guns:

"To the devil with your medicines," he said in exasperation, "I have already told you a hundred times that they would not do for me. I know my disease and my constitution better than you and all the physicians in the world. If I can perspire, and if I can open the scars on my thigh, I am cured. Yes, doctor, give me strength to go three or four leagues non-stop on horseback and do the same for fifteen or twenty successive days and you will see what health I enjoy."

And so they argued on until Napoleon, so convinced of the favourable results that would follow a sudden and violent change in his way of life, decided to put his belief to the test. He ordered his horse to be saddled and, followed by Noverraz and his groom, galloped for five or six miles round the old Longwood boundary. But, alas! the effect was not at all what he had expected; he didn't perspire and he felt distinctly the worse for wear.

Not one to give in easily, he behaved like a complete idiot and repeated the experiment another three or four times, returning feeling ever more clapped out. "My debilitated body can no longer deal with violent shocks, but I shall achieve my goal by moderate exercise." Unfortunately, his 'debilitated body' could no longer withstand even the moderate exercise of rides in his carriage which made him feel horribly sick.

During the next week Napoleon's health went rapidly downhill and, distressed at the way his patient was deteriorating in front of his very eyes, Antommarchi became extremely emotional and took to his bed with a violent fever. But after ten days with no physician Napoleon decided enough was enough and summoned his doctor to his bedside. Making an effort, Antommarchi pulled himself together and went to the Emperor's room where he found him in bed complaining of intolerable pain in the left side of his abdomen which radiated widely.

February 20 was another bad day with vomiting and loss of appetite. Even though he said he felt thoroughly worn out, he still wanted to talk.

"Well, doctor, will it be soon," he asked, death in the forefront of his mind.

"No, Sire, your illness is settling down."

"As always, doctor! When will you tire of telling me I'll recover?"

"When your health is restored."

"In that case you'll be making promises for a very long time to come."

"No, it will be sooner than Your Majesty might think. Your health, though, would benefit from taking the waters at a spa."

"Do you really believe they [the English] would acknowledge that? And if they did, a refusal would bring them into the open. It would be like admitting to my assassination. Poor *capo-corsino*! You do not understand them."

"But surely Sire, when your health demands it, when your doctor advises it, it would be inhuman to forbid it."

"Precisely!"

During the last days of February and the first half of March Napoleon ate little and that mostly light snacks of soup or broth, fresh eggs and a glass of well-diluted claret. He did, however, occasionally ask for more substantial meals such as roast lamb and fried potatoes, but would scarcely touch them.

Although he had enough to worry about on his own account, Napoleon still concerned himself with the fate of his own people on the island. Thus he noticed that the Abbé Buonavita was always unwell and, although his services were appreciated, they were not essential. Home he should go, and with a pension of three thousand francs. Antommarchi was told to see him safely on board his ship at Jamestown and make sure he had everything he might need on the long voyage. This provided an excellent opportunity for Antommarchi to slip the Abbé a letter for Chevalier Colonna informing Madame Mère of the Emperor's latest condition. It was dated the seventeenth of March, 1821:

> "In my letter to you of the eighteenth of July,1820, I spoke of the chronic hepatitis under which His Majesty is labouring. That disease, endemic in these latitudes, appeared, nevertheless, to yield to the action of our remedies: I obtained some amelioration; but relapses occurred, and since then there have been continual abrupt changes which completely destroy the effect of such treatment as has been given. The Emperor's situation is growing steadily worse; the

hepatic functions are no longer performed, and those of the digestive organs are completely suspended. His Majesty is now reduced to such a state, that he can only feed upon liquid substances, which do not, as it were, require to be digested; and it is not even certain that these reach the stomach, since they are rejected almost immediately after they have been taken.

"Such being the case, and in order to discharge myself from all responsibility, I declare to you, to all the imperial family, and to the whole world, that the disease under which the Emperor is labouring is an effect of the nature of the climate, and that the symptoms it exhibits are of the most serious kind.

"Art is unavailing against the continued action of the air we breathe; and if the English Government does not hasten to remove Napoleon from this destructive atmosphere, I grieve to say that His Majesty will soon be no more.

"The English newspapers constantly repeat that the Emperor's health is good: but do not believe them; the event will prove whether those from whom they receive their intelligence are sincere or well informed.

"Your friend,

F. ANTOMMARCHI."

When he got back to Longwood, he was quizzed by a concerned Napoleon about the boat and its crew; he was able to reassure him on most points, but what he could not answer was how the Abbé would be received in Rome.

"At any rate," said the Emperor, "they owe it to me to treat him well; for, after all, without me what would have become of the Church?" This was yet another allusion to Napoleon's restoration of Christianity after its banning by the Revolution.

As he laid out so clearly in his letter, the Emperor's disease was becoming more serious by the day and a deeply worried Antommarchi wanted a second opinion but he knew Napoleon would refuse to see an English physician. His perplexity was increased when the Governor offered the services of a newly-arrived physician "whose skill was incomparable and who could cure every disorder". (I never discovered the identity of this latter-day Hippocrates.) Antommarchi duly reported the offer to the Emperor.

"So as to introduce another Baxter to be his spy and concoct false bulletins! Does the Governor still need to disabuse Europe? Or is he already thinking of the autopsy? I will not have any man who is in communication with him."

Antommarchi made no comment but waited till Napoleon came off the boil. He then hazarded a few words on the need for a consultation.

"A consultation! What would that achieve? You all work in the dark; another physician would see no more than you what is going on in my body. And if he pretended he could, I should call him a quack and lose what little confidence I still have left in the children of Hippocrates. Besides, who should I consult?"

But the Emperor hadn't cooled down and Antommarchi had to wait still longer before again resuming his argument. "You persist," said Napoleon in a kindly voice, "well, I give my consent. Go and consult with the physician you consider the most skilful on the island."

And so, wasting no time, a greatly relieved Antommarchi had his horse saddled and rode out of Longwood on the Deadwood trail to talk to Archibald Arnott, senior surgeon of the 20th Regiment of Foot, the doctor who had conducted him round the island's hospitals.

After Antommarchi had recited the leading symptoms to him, Arnott's main concern was the state of the bowels since he believed they needed to be kept far more open than was the case. (All was well with Arnott's world if his patients could keep their bowels well and truly open.) His first recommendation, therefore, was that

Antommarchi should give whatever purgative Napoleon would accept. Secondly, he advised that a large blister should be raised in the region of the stomach; thirdly, he thought frequent sprinkling of the forehead with vinegar would be soothing; and, finally, he wanted Napoleon to have fizzy saline drinks.

When Antommarchi got back to Longwood, the fever had decreased and a couple of enemas were of further benefit. The Emperor was, however, decidedly unimpressed by Arnott's recommendations: "That is what the English do," he said and refused to have anything to do with them.

Two days later, on March 28, an early morning enema produced an abundant evacuation of thick, glutinous slimy matter. Since Napoleon's abdomen was tense and painful, Antommarchi suggested a mild purgative, but as soon as he heard the word, Napoleon stretched himself out, let his head fall forward and feigned sleep. Antommarchi, nevertheless, continued with all his usual arguments. When he sensed they were coming to an end, Napoleon gave a deep sigh, "What were you saying, doctor?" So Antommarchi began again and Napoleon went back to sleep again. At length Antommarchi knew he was beaten, and left. During the rest of the day the Emperor showed some improvement and ate more than usual.

The evidence of disease in the abdomen was progressing rapidly and again Antommarchi did his best to persuade Napoleon to take his medicines, but with no better luck than previously.

"*Quod scriptum, scriptum.* Can you doubt, doctor, that everything that happens is already recorded; that the hour of our death is predetermined and nothing we can do can change that." Antommarchi contradicted him and was sent "to the devil with your drugs."

But before he could reach his room he was called back to have Napoleon tell him that, in future, he would behave more respectfully towards medicine – even though the very idea was repugnant to him. Then, turning to Madame Bertrand, he asked:

"How do you manage to take all those pills the doctor is constantly prescribing for you?"

"I take them without thinking about it," she answered, "and I advise Your Majesty to do the same." He then put the question to Montholon and to his valets, all of whom had been indisposed at some time, and from all he received the same answer.

"Am I, then, to be the only one who rebels against medicine? I will no longer be so. Treat me!" And Antommarchi gave him ten grains of rhubarb which had the desired purgative effect.

Napoleon's worsening condition meant that if he wasn't actually in bed, he remained in his room. This made the orderly officer's task of confirming his presence twice a day a virtual non-starter. In Lowe's jittery state, the passing of a few days without a report gave him an almighty fright because he believed he had been hoodwinked while Napoleon was spirited away. So, with his staff in tow, he took off for Longwood where, riding round the building, he could see nothing to give his troubled mind some rest. Captain Engelbert Lutyens (the orderly officer) was consequently threatened with the severest of punishments if he failed to satisfy himself that General Bonaparte was still at Longwood.

In such an impossible situation, Lutyens appealed to Montholon and Marchand, who rose to the challenge. They would think up something to prevent the Emperor having the slightest suspicion that the Governor's agent was present.

Napoleon's bedroom was on the ground floor with its windows low enough for anyone outside to see what was happening inside. It was one of Napoleon's numerous enemas that provided the solution. Marchand placed the commode opposite the window while Antommarchi and Montholon took up station on either side. Marchand then adjusted the curtains a little as if he wanted to look at something in the garden. Lutyens, waiting outside, saw and made his report.

But the Governor was still not satisfied and declared that if on the next day or, at the latest, the day after, Lutyens had not been allowed to see the General properly, he would come to Longwood with his staff and, regardless of the consequences, force his way in. He turned a deaf ear to all Montholon's warnings of the effect this would have on Napoleon's feelings and actions. But it was of little concern to Lowe whether the prisoner lived or died; his duty was to ensure the security of his person, and that duty he would fulfil.

Mercifully, the arrival of Arnott at Longwood to begin his attendance on Napoleon broke the deadlock. He was acceptable to both sides.

* * *

And now, *mon ami(e)*, you understand that Napoleon was a very sick man and getting no better. The symptoms and signs of his progressing ill-health over the past few months consisted largely of variations on an established theme, all the while building towards an unhappy conclusion which Antommarchi clearly foresaw unless the Emperor was moved to a healthy climate. Most notably, the gastric ulcer leaked again, but fortunately again sealed itself off. And in the midst of all his mental and physical turmoil, Napoleon was still able to show concern for others, as when Antommarchi cut the back of his hand, and when he sent the Abbé Buonavita home with a pension.

~25~
Arnott: a second opinion

(APRIL 1 – 26, 1821)

Dr Archibald Arnott was the only doctor to attend Napoleon and emerge unscathed. Apart from the fact that he was in attendance for only four weeks, his good fortune may be attributed to his 'Englishness' – although Scottish by birth, he had been surgeon to the 20th Regiment of Foot since 1799 and had won ten clasps to his Peninsular Medal. He did indeed feel a degree of Englishness, since he was proud of the fact that "*no* other English medical person saw him [Napoleon] in his death-bed sickness." But whatever the case, he was afflicted with the English conviction that no matter what ailed Napoleon, the climate of St Helena had nothing to do with it. His letter to Lowe after Napoleon's death is an absolute gem of its kind:

> "The climate of St. Helena I consider healthy; the air is pure and temperate, and Europeans enjoy their health, and retain the vigour of their constitution, as in their native country.
>
> "It is true, I have witnessed a great deal of disease in St. Helena, but that viz. dysentery, and other acute diseases of the abdominal viscera, prevailed among the troops. The sickness of English soldiers, however, is not always a criterion of the insalubrity of a colony; their habits are very different from those of the higher ranks of life; they do not take that care of themselves which is so indispensable in a tropical climate to guard against atmospherical vicissitudes; they are also prone to intemperance, which renders the system more susceptible of disease; . . . I can therefore safely assert, that any one

of temperate habits, who is not exposed to much bodily exertion, night air, and atmospherical changes, as a soldier must be, may have as much immunity from disease in St. Helena as in Europe; and I may therefore further assert, that the disease of which Napoleon Bonaparte died was *not* the effect of climate."

Arnott knew which side his bread was buttered. He had seen what had happened to O'Meara and Stokoe and, after twenty-six years' army service, he was not about to let the same thing happen to him. Also, he made a pretty good job of batting for both sides.

On April 1 Antommarchi was again seriously concerned about Napoleon's health and without difficulty got his permission to call Arnott to Longwood. At 10.30pm Arnott was waiting in the orderly officer's quarters when Antommarchi came to collect him. He was led through the labyrinth of dimly lit passages to Napoleon's bedroom which was in total darkness. Napoleon was either drawing attention to the point he had made a week earlier that all physicians worked in the dark or – and this would not have been out of character – he wanted to enjoy the private joke of making Arnott *un poisson d'Avril*; it was April 1 after all! Anyway, Montholon took charge and guided him to the imperial bedside and formally introduced him.

Arnott politely enquired after the Emperor's state of health and the nature of his complaints. He then made a excellent job of examining a patient he could not see: the pulse was tranquil, the temperature moderate (determined by touch) and the skin slightly sweaty. Napoleon was enthusiastically complaining about his belly but Arnott could discover no tension or hardness. Under the circumstances, he did not prescribe anything and was dismissed with the injunction to return at nine o'clock next morning.

At 9am Arnott visited a patient he was able to see. He found him to be thoroughly depressed with a pulse rate of 76 per minute, a normal temperature (by touch), a heavily coated tongue and a remarkably pale complexion. He was still complaining of his stomach, specifically of a gnawing pain, and of feeling constantly sick with episodes of vomiting. He admitted to being seriously constipated and told Arnott that he seldom had his bowels open without the assistance of an enema. Napoleon took the opportunity right from the offset to make it plain to his new doctor that he strongly objected to taking any medicines whatsoever. Indeed, he said, his stomach was so irritable, that he was rarely able to keep anything, be it food or medicine, down.

After the customary argument with their patient the doctors managed to get him to agree to take a purgative in pill form. Arnott also recommended a diet of jellies and such easily digestible foods as the stomach would accept.

Thus, happily, Arnott's and Antommarchi's findings and recommendations for management were in general agreement, with both doctors laying stress on the importance of keeping the bowels open. The single point on which they parted company was the influence of the climate. Neither was prepared to change his mind: the one because of intellectual honesty; the other because of his buttered bread.

Arnott continued to live at the Deadwood camp and rode in twice a day or as required. When he visited that evening, it was really no surprise that Napoleon hadn't taken the purgative pills. So, as he hadn't had his bowels open for forty-eight hours he was given an enema the result of which was hardly worth the effort.

After a tolerable night with a good deal of sleep, Napoleon's pulse rate was unchanged at 76 per minute; his temperature was 96 degrees Fahrenheit (taken with a clinical thermometer, an unusual instrument at that time); his skin was clammier than usual; his spirits were low, and he felt drowsy. He told Arnott he could eat nothing even though his stomach was comfortable and he would like some wine; Arnott allowed him a little claret. His valets were instructed to continue to offer him jellies, light puddings, milk and other mild drinks. For what it was worth, he was urged, yet again, to take any form of purgative he found acceptable, but, said Arnott, "there was really so much apathy and indifference about our patient, that our arguments made no impression on him."

As Antommarchi (the two doctors had attended together) was leaving the Emperor's bedroom, he bumped into a worried Thomas Reade who was desperately anxious to see Napoleon installed in the new Longwood house which had been specially built for him – it would make good propaganda. Reade was amazed at Antommarchi for allowing him to stay in old Longwood and be suffocated in such ill-ventilated, unhealthy rooms when a magnificent new building awaited his arrival. Oh my god! I couldn't believe it. At last the English were admitting to the appallingly unhealthy living conditions at Longwood.

"I understand!" Antommarchi was incensed. "Killed in a hut, he must be seen to die in a palace. The combination is typically English! I will not lend myself to it. Try someone else." And Reade did.

That evening, before they had even reached the bedside, Arnott started to expound on the advantages of moving to the new house. Napoleon listened without saying a word. After a few minutes thought, he turned to Antommarchi:

"Is that your opinion, doctor?"

"No, Sire, your fever is too violent. To move you to another house could have the most serious consequences."

"You have heard," he said to Arnott. "Well! we shall say no more about it." Arnott, nevertheless, did his best to keep the argument going, but the Emperor simply turned a deaf ear and that was that. Napoleon remained in his 'hut'.

And so the days progressed. On April 10 his stomach was very irritable and his strength was failing. "The fever is past," he announced, "and I am now back to the state in which I have been languishing for the past eight months, which is to say, great weakness and lack of appetite, and then," he put his hand on his right side and looked at Arnott, " then there is the liver." Arnott took the hint and examined the region. Finding nothing out of the ordinary, he told Napoleon, "I do not find any disease of the liver," and then, basing his remark on the symptoms in general, went on, "but perhaps there might be a little want of action in it." (Actually, this is not as contradictory as might at first sight appear.)

Napoleon was totally unconvinced and showed it; he shook his head with a sardonic smile and said "So be it, doctor. I am obliged to you for the hope you try to give me. Now go."

On April 11, Antommarchi treated the Emperor's icy cold legs with fomentations. "No," said Napoleon, "the disease is not there. You will find it in the stomach, in the liver. You have no remedies capable of slaking the fire that rages within me!"

Arnott made yet another attempt to persuade him that his liver was sound.

"Yes, it must be so," Napoleon retorted, "since such is Hudson's decree!"

Although his bowels were still refusing to perform on their own, Napoleon stubbornly refused to take any opening medicines. "I shall take no more of them," he said to Antommarchi, "I prefer enemas – they are the simplest and most efficacious of remedies. The English," he added with a grin, "are ashamed to use them; but I am not so squeamish and submit to necessity. Doctor, you ought to marry."

Without warning , Napoleon had changed the subject.

"I must arrange a marriage for you."

"For me, Sire?"

"Yes, you."

Antommarchi remained silent, unsure what Napoleon was getting at.

"You are too warm, too quick. You need something to calm you down. So marry an Englishwoman; her iced blood will temper the fire that drives you, and you will become less stubborn."

"My one object is to do the best for Your Majesty; I have no intention of doing anything that might displease you."

"I know that, doctor, so from now on I shall be more obedient. Give me the medicine."

He took it and swallowed it in a single draught. "When a man," he said, " has been guilty of irreverence towards Galen, it is thus that the sin must be expiated." But, as always, his obedience lasted for only so long as it suited him.

Three days later, feeling better, Napoleon was discussing British military commanders with Arnott and praising, in particular, Marlborough.

"Does your regiment possess a copy of his campaigns?"

"I think not," Arnott replied.

"Well, I have a copy which I am glad to offer to that gallant regiment. Take it and put it in their library as a gift from me." But when the Governor caught Arnott leaving Longwood with the *Life of Marlborough* tucked under his arm he refused to let him put it in the library. Arnott, scared that the book "would give him the plague", lost no time in handing it over to Lutyens who did catch a dose of the plague: when the Governor learnt what had happened, he was dismissed from his post. However, he wasn't unduly upset as he had already applied to resign from his duties as orderly officer – creeping around after emperors on commodes was not his favourite pastime!

On the fifteenth Napoleon shut himself up with Montholon and Marchand for the whole afternoon while he drew up his will, a task he found extremely exhausting. "My preparations are made, doctor," he said when he next saw Antommarchi, "I am going; it is all over with me." Antommarchi tried hard to reassure him that his case was not desperate, but Napoleon interrupted him. "No more illusion, I know the truth and am resigned."

Over the following days, when he felt strong enough, he made lists of all his possessions, adding a number of codicils instructing how everything should be distributed.

On April 25, after a very bad night with incessant exhausting vomiting, his pulse rate was 82 per minute. An enema had small result. The vomiting continued throughout the day with his stomach rejecting everything swallowed. Noticing that when the bowels were open, the vomiting was less violent, Arnott managed to persuade Napoleon to take a full dose of mixture of magnesium sulphate. It emptied the bowels all right but, alas, without the usual favourable effect on the vomiting.

That evening, when Antommarchi was out of the room, Napoleon rebelled and ordered fruit and wine to be brought; he ate a biscuit, drank champagne, asked for a plum and grabbed some grapes. When Antommarchi returned, Napoleon burst out laughing but everything was taken away and the servant severely ticked off. But the damage was done: the fever returned and the Emperor was delirious until three in the morning when he fell asleep.

* * *

And now, *mon ami(e)*, you understand that Napoleon was not much longer for this world. Antommarchi was so worried that he called in Dr Arnott who agreed with him on most important matters except the influence of the St Helena climate. For the previous six or seven months Napoleon had had a poor appetite and the light diet he had been taking did little to sustain him; more recently, what he did consume was as often as not brought straight back. Despite the care lavished upon him by his devoted staff, Napoleon had become quite seriously malnourished and, largely by virtue of the persistent vomiting, dehydrated.

~26~
'Fast hastening to his grave"

(APRIL 27 – MAY 5, 1821)

The Emperor had had a very restless night, vomiting a lot and dropping off only at daybreak. At 8am, with both doctors at his bedside, he had a violent attack of retching and vomiting half-filling the bowl with a very offensive dark-coloured fluid resembling coffee-grounds. He had been bleeding into his stomach and the gastric juices had begun to digest the blood, hence its altered appearance. This vomiting continued until 3.30pm when he mercifully fell asleep. In the evening he was more comfortable, free from pain, but feeling low and exhausted. Although his bowels had not been opened for forty hours, he stubbornly refused any sort of treatment, even an enema. He rejected out of hand the suggestion that a blister be raised over his stomach. Eventually, in sheer desperation to be left alone, he agreed to have a warm stimulant aromatic plaster laid on his abdomen.

Between five and six o'clock, he took a little food which he managed to keep down, and then in the evening he at last agreed to leave his small, poorly ventilated bedroom and move into the drawing room. When he realized his valets were preparing to carry him, he remonstrated, "No, you may do that when I am dead. For the present it will be enough for you to support me."

At the end of the day Antommarchi commented, "Total debility: death has already claimed him; he is fast hastening to his grave."

On April 28, after another very bad night, there was more coffee-ground vomiting but this time with the addition of traces of fresh blood. His pulse was extremely weak and its rate varied between 84 and 90 per minute; his temperature (by touch) was decidedly subnormal. At about seven o'clock he had some soup, a fresh egg and a finger biscuit dunked in a little claret. At 8am, speaking calmly and with complete composure, he gave Antommarchi his instructions:

> "After my death, which cannot be far off, I want *you* to open my body. Also, and I insist on this, you will promise that no English medical man shall touch me. If, though, the assistance of one becomes absolutely necessary, Dr Arnott is the only one you have permission to call upon. I further wish that you will take my heart, put it in spirits of wine and take it to Parma to my dear Marie Louise. You will tell her that I loved her tenderly, that I have never stopped loving her, and you will tell her everything you have seen, everything concerning my situation and my death.
>
> "I particularly ask you to examine my stomach carefully, and to make a precise and detailed report of the state in which you find it and to give it to my son. . . . When I am no more you will go to Rome; you will see my mother and my family and will tell them everything about my predicament, my disorder and my death on this sad and unhappy rock. You will tell them that the great Napoleon breathed his last in a most deplorable state, deprived of everything except of himself and his glory. Tell them that, with his dying breath, he bequeathed all the horror and disgrace of his last moments to the reigning houses of Europe."

The fever suddenly left him at 10am and, although utterly exhausted, he continued to talk, albeit incoherently. At midday he had a little to eat only to have it returned a few hours later mixed with more coffee-ground vomitus which did, however, bring him some relief.

That night Napoleon again had little sleep and for most of the time was delirious and talking incessantly. Towards morning of the twenty-ninth he was beset by a violent attack of hiccups due to the uraemia of incipient kidney failure. In its turn, this attack brought on more coffee-ground vomiting. Nevertheless, when he awoke at midday, he was sensible and composed and had some vermicelli soup, a fresh egg and a little claret. At some time during the night, in a raving fit, he had torn the aromatic plaster from his stomach. As it had had little or no effect, Antommachi suggested replacing it with a blister. This he was permitted to do, but so exhausted were the Emperor's bodily functions, that it failed to appear for twenty-one hours.

During the night Antommarchi applied two more blisters, one to the inside of each thigh. Napoleon slept for a few hours then, towards morning, lay awake, quiet and composed. He had vomited several times, but not so copiously and not of so dark a colour; he had also again been stricken with hiccups for a couple of hours. At noon he had a few more spoonfuls of vermicelli soup and another fresh egg. At 3pm the fever increased, to ease towards evening, but between nine and ten it increased again; he was agitated; the hiccups returned; breathing became difficult, and there were spasmodic risings from the stomach, accompanied by a sense of suffocation. He salivated a lot and there was an icy coldness all over his body. From time to time his pulse became imperceptible. He rallied towards 11.30pm.

On May 1 Napoleon was much worse. His pulse rate approached 100 per minute; his temperature was felt to be subnormal and his skin was damp and clammy. He continued hiccupping and vomiting. Towards midday he improved, but it couldn't last and in the afternoon he relapsed again, becoming delirious and talking incoherently. An enema produced a copious evacuation. During the day he ate two finger biscuits and drank only a little claret.

At noon on May 2 Antommarchi gave him an anodyne mixture of orange-flower water and a few drops of tincture of opium and ether. Towards 1pm he ate two finger biscuits dunked in diluted claret.

With the end approaching, a change was made in the night-time arrangements. Hitherto, Bertrand, Montholon, Antommarchi, Marchand and St-Denis (Ali) had taken it upon themselves to sit up in turns with their Emperor. However, as he could not abide the light, they had to lift and care for him in total darkness. Adding to their concern, they were now all extremely tired so, when the members of the French staff at Longwood begged to have a share in these duties, they were welcomed with sighs of relief.

On May 3 Napoleon awoke at 3am, restless and anxious with a pulse rate of 100 per minute. As the night came to an end, the hiccupping grew more violent and distressing. At 8.45 he enjoyed the yolk of an egg and the usual couple of finger biscuits with a little claret.

At noon he relapsed and at 2pm Abbé Vignali administered the last rites. Then, even though his symptoms were gathering force, he talked quite rationally about his achievements for France and what he had had to leave undone.

As the afternoon wore on Arnott felt it absolutely essential to free his bowels by whatever means and suggested giving 10 grains of calomel without the patient's knowledge. Antommarchi opposed the plan on the grounds that the Emperor was too weak and would be weakened further to no good purpose. However, the Governor unwittingly stepped in by ordering the Longwood doctors to hold a consultation with Dr Thomas Shortt, Principal Medical Officer on the island, and Dr Charles Mitchell, surgeon on HMS *Vigo*, currently flag ship on the St Helena station.

They met in Antommarchi's apartment where he outlined the clinical picture. This, however, did not satisfy them as they naturally wanted to see the patient for themselves. On Antommarchi's assurance that this was a hopeless ambition, they resigned themselves to agreeing with Arnott. The 10 grains of calomel were accordingly administered at 6pm.

At 7pm, the Emperor was offered a few spoonfuls of *sabaillon* (white wine and sugar) which he could swallow only with the help of water. Violent hiccupping ensued. When the calomel was still without effect at ten o'clock, the British doctors wanted to give another dose, but this time Antommarchi dug his heels in and refused to allow it, regardless of etiquette. His judgment was proved correct when, at 11pm the bowels began to clear themselves with five abundant evacuations of fetid tarry stools (evidence of the bleeding at the upper end of the alimentary tract). Napoleon was left in a state of complete collapse and suffering severe difficulty with breathing. There was little change during the rest of the night.

The fourth of May dawned with the storm that is an obligatory accompaniment of supernatural cataclysms and the deaths of heroes. Antommarchi described it most sympathetically:

> "The weather was frightful; the rain fell in torrents, and the wind threatened to destroy everything. The willow under which Napoleon usually sat to enjoy the fresh air could not withstand the blast; the trees in our garden plantations were torn up by their roots and lay scattered around; a single gumwood tree was still standing until a whirlwind had it in its grasp and laid it prostrate in the mud. It seemed that none of the things the Emperor had valued were to survive him."

Napoleon continued to refuse all medicines and only with difficulty could he be enticed into taking a little cold broth. He did, however, drink a large quantity of the orange-flower-water mix, which was a mistake as it produced violent intestinal colic. He was hiccupping incessantly and suffering painful spasms in the upper part of his abdomen and over the stomach. His bowels were open three more times but by now he was unconscious, unaware of what was happening and showing the typical Hippocratic facies of imminent death. Towards evening the fever increased and he salivated excessively.

He remained unconscious throughout the night until 5am when he began vomiting coffee-grounds; his bowels opened involuntarily with violent pains in the abdomen.

"The clock struck half-past five," reported Antommarchi, "and Napoleon was delirious, speaking with difficulty, and uttering words disjointedly and inarticulately; amongst others we heard 'Head . . . army,' and these were the last he uttered, for they had no sooner passed his lips than he lost the power of speech."

He developed severe difficulty in breathing and total loss of muscular movement; his eyes were staring; his pulse was feeble, intermittent and scarcely palpable in the carotid and axillary arteries; its rate varied between 102 and 112 per minute. After a while he rallied and began sighing deeply; his breathing had become slow, stertorous and intermittent – indicative of advancing left ventricular heart failure. His vital organs were packing up one by one: his liver, his kidneys and now his heart and lungs.

Madame Bertrand, who refused to leave the bedside, sent first for her daughter, Hortense, and then for her three sons. They had not seen Napoleon for close on two months and as they filed in their eyes filled with tears. Falling to their knees, they grasped his hands and smothered them with those tears. It was all too much for young Napoleon Bertrand who simply fainted and had to be carried into the garden. The other children were allowed a few minutes more before they too were led outside.

So that nothing should be seen to have been left undone – despite the fact that their patient was moribund – Arnott and Antommarchi set to work with a will; they both realized that if they didn't display all that medicine had to offer, no matter how hopeless, they would be in line for a gubernatorial tongue lashing. They placed a blister over the sternum and one on each thigh; two large mustard plasters on the soles of the feet; and warm fomentations with a bottle filled with hot water on the abdomen – all without effect. Antommarchi also moistened his lips which, had any sensibility remained, was the kindest gesture of them all.

The signs gathered momentum until, at eleven minutes before

six o'clock on the fifth of May, 1821, the Emperor Napoleon lay dead.

* * *

And now, *mon ami(e)*, you understand the manner of Napoleon's death. It had been inevitable for at least the past eight days and, dominating the clinical picture, were the signs that the vital organs were rapidly failing.

~27~
Post-mortem

(MAY 5, 1821 – APRIL 3, 1838)

So, *mon ami(e)*, Napoleon Bonaparte is no more. But are you any further ahead with knowing the cause of his death? Many people would hesitate until they knew the outcome of the post-mortem, but this will not be as trustworthy as you might think, for two main reasons. First, pathology was in a pretty primitive state and, as I shall emphasize in a moment, not all diseases that may afflict the stomach had yet been identified. And second, unless the offending tissue can be examined under the microscope the differential diagnosis in Napoleon's case between gastric cancer and gastric ulcer is impossible – and I do mean impossible – unless, of course, the stomach still resides in a suitable condition in its silver container in the coffin in Les Invalides, Paris, and permission could be obtained for the examination!

Nevertheless, in my opinion the clinical histories obtained by O'Meara and, in particular, by Antommarchi (because the disease developed during his watch) were reliable enough to bring the scales down in favour of gastric ulcer.

Before the post-mortem could begin a number of formalities had to be completed. Six hours had already passed, during which the French staff paid their respects, before Antommarchi had him shaved and his body washed and placed on another bed. Overnight, at the request of Montholon, it was Arnott who watched over the body.

Meantime, the executors were looking into their responsibilities regarding two of the codicils to the Emperor's will. One concerned a legacy to the members of his household and the distribution of alms to the poor of St Helena. The other was in two parts, the first of which read: "It is my wish that my ashes may rest on the banks of the Seine, among the French people, whom I loved so well."

The Governor was duly informed of the contents of the two documents and reacted true to form: The body was to remain on the island; England held it and would not give it up. That part of the will was completely inadmissible. He was utterly opposed to it. The executors tried their best to make him change his mind. But no, "the body of Napoleon is to remain on St Helena, and there it *will* remain." They invoked humanity, the respect due to the dead, but right vanishes before might, as Antommarchi expressed it, and all that could be done was to adopt the course of the weak – to protest and obey. And, indeed, this was the course pursued.

The spot chosen for the burial, the secluded Geranium Valley (otherwise known as Sane Valley) about a mile-and-a-half from Longwood, caused no dissension. Although Napoleon had seen the place only once, he spoke of it and the soothing waters of its spring quite fondly. Lowe may indeed have held the order to retain the body of Bonaparte, but where this body was buried was to him a matter of supreme indifference.

The next morning, once all this had been settled, the Governor galloped off to Longwood attended by his staff, the members of the island Council, Brigadier John Pine-Coffin (who, in August, 1820, had succeeded Sir George Bingham), Admiral Robert Lambert, the Marquis de Montchenu, all the physicians and surgeons on the island and three naval captains, one of whom was Captain Frederick Marryat, in command of the *Beaver*, and author of *The Children of the New Forest*, *Peter Simple* and other memorable (in their day) novels. Lowe's main objective was to make absolutely certain, by his own inspection, that Napoleon really was dead, and that the corpse before him really was that of Napoleon Bonaparte.

He also wanted the post-mortem to be performed immediately, but he had to wait until the death mask had been taken.

* * *

The post-mortem was conducted on the afternoon of May 6 in the presence of Bertrand, Montholon and Marchand (the three executors), Sir Thomas Reade, Doctors Shortt, Arnott, Mitchell, Livingstone, Henry and Rutledge, Abbé Vignali, St Denis (Ali) and a few staff officers. Madame Bertrand may also have been in the room. As requested by Napoleon the dissection was carried out by Antommarchi – and anyway, he was the only experienced morbid anatomist on the island.

But before I tell you about the post-mortem, it is vitally important that you are clear in your mind about one critical fact in the history of gastric pathology: Gastric ulcer was not described until ten or more years after Napoleon's death. So, as far as Antommarchi – and all the other doctors – were concerned there was no such disease as gastric ulcer. Gastric ulcer, as we understand the disease today, simply did not exist for them. Therefore, any nasty-looking lesion in the stomach *was* cancer; there was just no possibility that it could be anything else. When Antommarchi examined Napoleon's stomach, what he saw and what, in his mind, he was describing *was* gastric cancer.

Antommarchi may well have carried out the post-mortem, but his description did not become the official report; indeed, it was not published until 1825 when it appeared in his *Mémoires*. As well as these two reports, however, there was yet another which was prepared in 1823 by Walter Henry. Neither Henry nor the compilers of the official report sing from Antommarchi's hymn sheet. Their motives for not doing so have to be suspect.

While Napoleon's head was being shaved – in keeping with his wish to have his hair distributed among the members of his family – Antommarchi made a number of observations and measurements. His first impression was that Napoleon was thinner than at their first meeting some eighteen months previously. His face and body were pale, but without looking cadaverous. His eyes were closed as if he were deeply asleep, while a sardonic smile hovered around his mouth.

Henry was more lyrical: "The face presented a remarkably placid expression, indicative of mildness and even sweetness of disposition, which afforded a most striking contrast with the active life and moral character of the Deceased. The features were regular and even considered beautiful."

Napoleon's height from the top of his head to his heels was, in English measures, 5ft $6\frac{1}{2}$in; the circumference of his head was $20\frac{7}{8}$ in; the forehead was high, the temples slightly depressed and the sinciput (front part of the head) wide and very strongly defined.

Other bodily features noted by Antommarchi were: hair thin and of a light chestnut colour; neck rather short, but tolerably well proportioned; chest wide and well formed; abdomen considerably swollen and voluminous; hands and feet rather small; all other parts of the body were of normal proportions.

Now, I don't propose detailing everything that Antommarchi found during the dissection, since some things may be regarded as incidental and of no clinical significance and others may safely be attributed to the state of Napoleon's health during the preceding weeks and to the body having been lying for twenty-one hours. Although the upper lobe of the left lung was found to be studded with tubercles (pointing to infection in the distant past which was almost certainly asymptomatic) and several small tuberculous cavities (suggesting re-activation, possibly the consequence of his captivity and poor health on St Helena), it is the contents of the abdomen that are of the main interest to history.

When he opened the abdomen, Antommarchi found the peritoneal cavity to be distended by a large quantity of gas.The liver was hardened and swollen with blood. It was affected by chronic hepatitis. There were adhesions between it and the stomach and diaphragm. He described the gall-bladder as being filled and distended with extremely thick and clotted bile (he made no mention of gallstones). The official report says that except for the adhesions due to the disease in the stomach "no unhealthy appearance presented itself in the liver." It makes no mention at all of the gall-bladder. Henry, on the other hand, was prepared to commit himself: "The Gall Bladder was of proper size and structure containing no gall stones but the usual quantity of apparently healthy bile." He also stated that the liver was of natural size and perfectly healthy.

The stomach appeared to Antommarchi at first sight to be in a mostly healthy state with no trace of inflammation. But when he examined it more carefully, he discovered that, on the anterior surface towards the lesser curvature and three fingers' breadth from the pylorus, there was a very small and well circumscribed area of hardening. The stomach itself was penetrated through and through in the centre of this area. However, the hole was sealed off by the adhesions to the left lobe of the liver.

When he opened the stomach along its greater curvature, he was greeted by an acrid stench which came from a considerable quantity of 'matter' mixed with a lot of thick mucus resembling coffee-grounds. When this had been removed, an area of mucous membrane along the greater curvature was seen to be quite normal. However, nearly all the rest of the internal surface of the stomach was taken up by a 'cancerous' ulcer which extended along the lesser curvature from the cardiac orifice to within an inch or more of the pylorus.The right end of the stomach, an inch or so from the pylorus, was encircled by an indurated hardening about half an inch wide. The pyloric orifice itself was entirely normal.

The urinary bladder, empty and very contracted, contained a quantity of gravel mixed with a few small calculi. Numerous red plaques were scattered over the mucous membrane – all in all the walls of the bladder were not in a very healthy state.

To end proceedings, Antommarchi closed his incisions with a suture, washed the body and handed it over to Marchand who dressed it in the uniform of a Colonel of the Chasseurs de la Garde, wearing the cocked hat and with a crucifix at the breast.

The story of how the official British report came to be prepared is not exactly straightforward. It was signed by Thomas Shortt, MD, Physician and PMO; Archibald Arnott, MD, Surgeon 20th Regiment; Charles Mitchell, MD, Surgeon HMS *Vigo*; Francis Burton, MD, Surgeon 66th Regiment; and Matthew Livingstone, Surgeon Honourable East India Company.

Thomas Shortt had arrived on St Helena in December, 1820, and, as Principal Medical Officer assumed medical control of the island. As such, his was the responsibility of preparing the official post-mortem report. He said that a first draft had been drawn up by himself from notes taken, on his instructions, by Walter Henry, Assistant Surgeon 66th Foot, who was too junior to be a signatory. This first draft concluded with the observation that "the liver was perhaps a little larger than natural" and was signed only by Shortt, Arnott, Burton and Mitchell.

Livingstone had not been an original signatory as he had, for some reason, left the post-mortem before the end. Lowe smelt a rat, believing that Shortt had sent Livingstone away for reasons of his own. But as Superintendent of the East India Company's Medical Establishment on St Helena, he was Lowe's man and had to be a signatory. In Shortt's presence Lowe asked him whether he had noticed anything abnormal about the liver and, like a good establishment Englishman, Livingstone answered "No". The offending comment was accordingly crossed out (but remained perfectly legible); Shortt was not prepared to argue – he knew what had happened to Stokoe. However, he left a note on the draft (which was not destroyed) to the effect that this comment had been suppressed by order of Sir Hudson Lowe. It was vital to Lowe that there should not be the slightest hint anywhere that Napoleon had died from anything that could cast aspersions on the way the British had cared for him (i.e. involvement of the liver); cancer of the stomach was the ideal diagnosis.

So, the official report was re-written and signed again, but with Livingstone added to the previous signatories. In its final version it did, regrettably, establish the belief that Napoleon had died from *cancer* of the stomach. Not one of the five signatories had taken part in the dissection, they were simply among the gathering of observers.

Antommarchi's explanation of why he was not himself a signatory was that the next day, while he was watching the crowds at Napoleon's lying in state, Shortt, Mitchell and Burton had emerged from the orderly officer's quarters and had headed towards him. It had "suddenly occurred to them that it was their duty to frame the report: they had consequently written that report, and now brought it to me for my signature, which I refused to give." The reason for this, according to Rutledge, Assistant Surgeon, 20th Regiment, was that Bertrand refused to give permission for him to do so because the report did not call Napoleon the Emperor. (As in life, so in death.)

The official post-mortem report was included among Lowe's dispatches announcing the death of Napoleon which were sent to London on the evening of May 7 and arrived in England on July 4.

Henry's report has since attracted attention for all the wrong reasons. It was written at Lowe's request in 1823 by Henry from the notes he had made at the time. Much of what he wrote is, not unsurprisingly, an almost word-for-word repeat of the official document; there are, however, some intriguing differences and additions. For instance:

> "The whole surface of the body was deeply covered with fat. Over the sternum where, generally, the bone is very superficial, the fat was upwards of <u>an inch</u> deep, and an inch and a half, or perhaps two inches, on the Abdomen. The skin was noticed to be particularly white and delicate as were the hands and arms. Indeed the whole

body was slender and effeminate. There was scarcely any hair on the body and that of the head was thin, fine and silky. [The pubis much resembled the Mons Veneris in women.] The muscles of the Chest were small; the shoulders were narrow and the Hips wide."

"The Spleen, Pancreas and Intestines were sound. The Kidneys were imbedded in an immense quantity of fat. The left kidney was one third larger than the right – this enlargement appeared to have been congenital. [The Urinary Bladder was small and contained a few gritty particles. The Penis and Testicles were very small, and the whole Genital system seemed to exhibit a Physical cause for the absence of sexual desire and the chastity which had been stated to have characterized the Deceased.]"

The two sections of text within the square brackets were crossed out at the time but left eminently readable. Perhaps Henry may have considered he had gone a little too far but was still intent on heaping further ignominy on the fallen Emperor by making him out to have had an effeminate body and, generally, not to have been much of a man. But what an extraordinary contradiction for him to say that the whole body was slender and effeminate when he had just drawn attention to the whole surface of the body being deeply covered in fat. Henry was just trying too hard. However, he did not labour in vain as these two sections were to attract as much attention as if they had been part of the official report – and be believed. Surprised?

At the time of the centenary of the battle of Waterloo, the science of endocrinology was breaking out of its shell and the diagnostic possibilities it offered were exploited to breaking point. A Scottish physician, Leonard Guthrie, made hay with Henry's report, reckoning that the two passages were sufficient to justify the diagnosis of hypopituitarism – even though they had been crossed out? So persuasive was the argument that it was still seriously considered after the Second World War. And I wouldn't be surprised that if you asked around now you could find people who seriously believed that Napoleon suffered from deficiency of the pituitary gland. Quite a tribute to the power of Walter Henry's imagination!

But it's about time we returned to events after the post-mortem.

* * *

The first of these was the lying-in-state which took place on the seventh of May in Napoleon's bedroom. The body was lying on a small camp bed, covered with the dark blue cloak General Bonaparte had worn at the battle of Marengo. The feet and hands were exposed to view.

As Antommarchi was about to leave the room at its conclusion, he was approached by the Governor, "ever humane, compassionate, and sincere, he deplored the loss we had sustained." [I am fairly sure Antommarchi was being sarcastic when he said this, although, of course, the Governor could have been unable to contain the overwhelming relief he felt at having an almost intolerable burden lifted from his shoulders.] He said the loss was the more to be regretted as his Government was becoming more favourably disposed and "had ordered him to tell General Bonaparte that the moment was approaching when his liberty might possibly be restored; and that his Britannic Majesty would not be the last to hasten the end of his captivity." Lowe's information had come in a letter from Lord Bathurst.

But could humanity really have been about to prevail?

* * *

And what of Antommarchi? He sailed from St Helena on May 27, 1821, on board the supply ship, *Camel*; his fellow passengers included the Bertrand family, Count Montholon, Abbé Vignali and two hundred soldiers. They reached Portsmouth on July 31. Five days later he left for London where he appeared before a council of ministers to be questioned on the climate of St Helena.

Early in September he set off for Rome where, after some passport problems, he fulfilled the promises he had made to Napoleon regarding Madame Mère and the imperial family. On his way back to France he was detained a few days in Florence by some 'bizarre' claims made by Mascagni's heirs regarding the publication of his atlas and who owned the rights; these were not resolved. Back in Paris he found himself caught up in legal wrangles over Napoleon's will. When these were brought to a satisfactory conclusion in June, 1823, he happily resumed his studies – "they are preferable to arbitration and lawsuits."

These studies included the completion of his *Mémoires ou Les derniers momens de Napoléon* which was published in 1825. Six years later, inspired by the plight of the Polish people in their latest rising against Russia, he travelled to Warsaw to volunteer his services. He arrived on May 17, 1831, and was appointed to the newly-created post of Inspector-General of the Military Hospitals on the twenty-sixth. During June he wrote a creditable memoir on the cholera currently prevalent in the Warsaw hospitals. However, after the revolt of August 15, he realized that, with traitors scheming to hand Poland over to the Russians who were then closing in on Warsaw, he would be better off out of the unhappy country. Accordingly, he submitted his resignation which was accepted on the twenty-third.

He then lived in Paris until 1834 when he travelled to the United States of America. He practised for a while in New Orleans, presenting the city with a bronze copy of Napoleon's death mask and the instruments he had used at the post-mortem. (These can't be found; they were possibly lost during the Civil War.) But he couldn't settle down, going to Mexico and California before dying of yellow fever in Santiago, Cuba, on April 3, 1838, at the age of forty-nine. A sad and lonely end for a good doctor who simply was on the wrong side at the wrong time and has, for many historians, stayed there.

* * *

And now, *mon ami(e)*, you are aware that what I am going to tell you about the cause of Napoleon's death is my opinion, but it is an opinion based on the totality of the clinical picture as recorded by the doctors who cared for him, together with the report of one of those doctors, an experienced morbid anatomist, who performed the post-mortem. It is not based on a cherry-picking expedition through that picture to fit preconceived ideas.

The condition most apparent at the time of death was a simple gastric ulcer which had leaked and become sealed off six months earlier and had begun to bleed eight or nine days before the death. The post-mortem showed that he had indeed been suffering from a gastric ulcer and also from cholecystitis; the presence of gallstones was not recorded though the clinical history suggested that they might have been present. There was some liver pathology, possibly hepatitis. None of this was sufficient of itself to have been the cause of death, not even the bleed from the ulcer which may have been alarming but was not massive.

As you saw, Napoleon had become seriously malnourished and dehydrated, in consequence of which his kidneys had been unable to deal with the metabolic and electrolytic imbalance and had begun to fail. His heart and lungs were also showing signs of imminent failure. All of this has to be viewed against a backdrop of possible iron-deficiency anaemia and the likelihood of vitamin C deficiency.

You were looking at a man dying of multi-system failure. None of the identifiable diseases was directly responsible for the moment of death.

And so at last, *mon ami(e)*, you have the answers to our two questions. I have said my goodbyes to Napoleon Bonaparte and now I bid farewell to you, trusting that you appreciate the significance of Miss Fanny Mitchell.

* * *

Should you feel inclined to check on my interpretation of the four doctors' journals, my references are:

O'Meara BE. (1822). *Napoleon in Exile; or, A Voice from St. Helena. The opinions and reflections of Napoleon on the important events of his life and government, in his own words.* 2 vols. 5th ed. London; Simpkin and Marshall. (First edition, also 1822.)

Stokoe J. (1902). *With Napoleon at St. Helena: Being the Memoirs of Dr. John Stokoe, Naval Surgeon. Translated from the French of Paul Frémeaux by Edith S. Stokoe.* London and New York; John Lane The Bodley Head.

Antommarchi F. (1825). *Mémoires du Docteur F. Antommarchi ou Les Derniers Momens de Napoléon.* 2 vols. Paris; Barrois. (Please note that the word is '*Momens*' and NOT '*Moments*' as almost invariably written.)

Antommarchi F. (1826). *Memoirs of the Last Two Years of Napoleon's Exile.* 2 vols. 2nd ed. London; Colburn. (First edition, 1825.)

Arnott A. (1822). *An Account of the Last Illness, Decease, and Post Mortem Appearances, of Napoleon Bonaparte. To which is added a letter from Dr. Arnott to Lieutenant-General Sir Hudson Lowe, K.C.B. &. giving a succinct statement of Napoleon Bonaparte's disease and demise.* London; Murray.

Index